Hope this helps

The Porcelain Doll:

My life with mental illness

by

Janet Knudsen

I came back!
Janet

DREAMCATCHER PUBLISHING
Saint John • New Brunswick • Canada

DreamCatcher Publishing acknowledges the support of the New Brunswick Arts Council.

Canadian Cataloguing in Publication Data

Knudsen, Janet - 1964

The Porcelain Doll (My life with mental illness)

ISBN - 1-894372-32-8
          1. Knudsen, Janet, 1964- 2. Manic-depressive persons--Rehabilitation. 3. Manic-depressive persons--Biography. I. Title.
          RC516.K58 2004   616.89'5'0092   C2004-901228-2

Editor: Yvonne Wilson

Typesetter: Chas Goguen

Cover Design: Dawn Drew, INK Graphic Design Services Corp.

Lily logo designed by Wanda Knudsen

Printed and bound in Canada

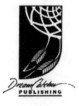

DREAMCATCHER PUBLISHING INC.
105 Prince William Street
Saint John, New Brunswick, Canada E2L 2B2
www.dreamcatcherbooks.ca

I dedicate this book

To God for His inspiration, guidance, direction, strength and love.

To my family whose love and encouragement are infinite:

Thank you to my mom, Charlotte, and my dad, Ben, for never losing hope. Without their love, I would not have gotten well. A special thank you to my mom for reading my book throughout the writing process, for offering suggestions and ideas, and for being the best mom a person could want.

Thank you to my sisters, Wanda, Julie and Tammy, who stood by me even though they did not understand my illness . . . God knows it could not have been easy.

Thank you to my brother-in-law Graham Bentley who visited me in the hospital countless times, who met me while I was sick, and who stuck around despite my illness.

Thank you to my brother-in-law Ryan Arsenault.

Thank you to my nephew Jordan David, who is a constant reminder that life is truly glorious, miraculous and full of wonder.

To Dr. Eric Taubner for his perseverance, dedication and caring for which I am eternally grateful.

To all members of the psychiatric profession including the dedicated doctors, nurses and researchers without whom I would not be well today.

To my university English teacher, Lois Armes Lawrence, PhD, who encouraged me to write and whose words of inspiration and encouragement remained with me. She gave freely of her time and knowledge and was one of my staunchest supporters.

To Carl Lotsberg, my guitar teacher and my friend, who contributed greatly to my wellness.

To Trevor Roy, my closest friend, whose beautiful piano playing was like a light in the darkness—a light that gave me hope and joy in my darkest hour.

To Glenn Orsak, MD, my longtime friend, who always said that I had a way with words.

To Denise Angerame, my first outside reader, who encouraged me throughout the long writing process and who always managed to say the right thing at the right time.

To Yvonne Wilson, my editor; Elizabeth Margaris, my publisher; and Chas Goguen, executive assistant, at DreamCatcher Publishing for believing in me and my book.

To Dawn Drew, my cover artist.

To all who suffer from mental illness. Never lose hope!

Acknowledgments

After the Gold Rush
© 1970 Neil Young
Cotillion Music Inc. &
Broken Arrow Music Corp.

Cotillion Music Inc.
C/O Warner Chappell Music Inc.
10585 Santa Monica Blvd.
Los Angeles, CA, 90025-4921
Phone: (310) 441-8600

Me and Bobby McGee
© 1969 Kris Kristofferson & Fred Foster
Combine Music Corp
Administered by EMI Blackwood Music Inc.

Solsbury Hill
© 1977 Peter Brian Gabriel
Real World Music Ltd.
Contact: publishing@realworld.co.uk

Sweetness and light
surround me

Sadness shows on my face

But God will restore my smile

Through His amazing grace

Preface

So . . . where do I begin? I suppose I could start with the great depression. More importantly, I could begin with why I am writing this tale, my story.

In 1993 my psychiatrist diagnosed me with manic depression. Addressing the term "manic depression" as opposed to the current moniker "bipolar illness" is a must for me. I think the latter term sounds like a weather report. Indeed, bipolar illness sounds benign. This nouveau politically correct name sugarcoats the severity of the illness. Manic depression is *not* like a cold. It does not disappear after a couple of weeks. It stays with you. No sooner do you think you are well than you are walking on the tightrope again, teetering on the edge of sanity. No matter which way you fall, into ecstasy or despair, you eventually hit the ground and are broken. When in the throes of manic depression, you *are* sick, you *are* crazy. So I believe the term "manic depression" far better conveys the nature of the illness, and that is the term I use.

When I am manic, I eventually become psychotic in that I suffer from paranoia, delusions and both auditory and visual hallucinations.

Psychiatrists distinguish between hallucinations and delusions. Hallucinations are false sensory perceptions; delusions are fixed, false ideas not rooted in either religious or cultural beliefs. To be psychotic is to suffer from hallucinations and/or delusions. I am diagnosed with psychotic mania, and not schizoaffective disorder or schizophrenia, because I do not cling to my delusions when I am well.

The possible side effects of my antipsychotic medication are obsessive-compulsive disorder, anxiety attacks and extreme fatigue. I guess when I do something, I do it in grand style. But suffering from all these illnesses, I feel I can write about them in an honest fashion. My goal, in short, is to describe what was going through my head. I feel both blessed and cursed in that I remember everything that happened around me and how my brain interpreted it. I am smoking a cigarette as I write this, my second in 15 minutes. I laughingly tell my doctor that the nicotine is a part of the chemical balance I currently enjoy. I started smoking during the great depression . . .

Chapter 1

Music is my life's love. As far back as I can remember, I have
loved music. I wanted to be a "singer lady" when I grew up. I wanted
to be the best guitar player in the world. Thank God for music. It
proved to be my savior, my sanity, my joy.

I was born September 18, 1964, in Montreal, Quebec, the
second of four girls. Despite a couple of moves, I considered myself
a Montrealer until the age of 17. The depression began when I was 10
years old. I resented being a child because I felt that I was not *free*.
Freedom, to me, was having a car and being allowed to go to adult-
only places. I hated being a child so much that I swore I would never
have children. The funny thing is that I have a wonderful, loving,
happy family. So why was I so depressed? Why did I feel life was a
curse from God, and death His gift?

One night at a bar, a man I knew asked me, "What was the last
good year?"

I immediately responded, "1974."

Later that night I wondered why I had answered so swiftly
and with such conviction. So I pondered childhood.

I was a happy, gregarious child who walked around the
neighborhood, blanket in hand. At age 3, I had a crush on the boy
who lived down the street and thought I would marry him when I

grew up. Indeed, I had already planned out my life. Starting nursery school in 1968 was thrilling.

I thought, "Now I will learn what grown-ups know."

Nursery school turned out to be nothing but playing, napping, milk and cookies coated in what I thought was red dye #5. I remember I enjoyed painting, but there were only two casels; so I hardly ever got to do that. Yeah, nursery school was a complete waste of my time. I learned how to read children's books the following summer. It was as though I were making up for lost time.

The words "lost time" give me pause. Throughout my life I have been plagued with the notion that I am supposed to do *something* and that I am running out of time. I have always tried to stay one step ahead of everyone. I feel like I have to do so. The something relates to God and His plan for me. It is typical of manic-depressives to be on a mission from God as I discovered when I met others so afflicted. The "mission from God" syndrome most often occurs when one is deeply manic, and I will address this topic in great detail later.

Kindergarten, too, was a waste of my precious time. My older sister Wanda was one grade ahead of me. Since I was not really learning anything at nursery school, I grilled Wanda daily to find out what she had learned in kindergarten and discovered that she had learned nothing that I did not already know. Leaving kindergarten with an ugly ashtray that I had made in art class and with the ability to beat two sticks together rhythmically that I had learned in music class, I felt I had lost another year of my life. Kindergarten did, however, ignite my interest in music.

The summer following kindergarten I started to sing. My dad let me play his wonderful eclectic collection of records on my child's record player, and every day I sang along with everyone from Nancy Sinatra to The Beatles. I memorized the lyrics easily. Nothing made me happier than singing.

I should mention that I was a television addict. My activities were usually indoors so I could watch the television and do whatever else I wanted to do at the same time. I did not much care for children's shows; talk shows and game shows were my favorites. As for cartoons, I preferred those with adult undertones. I wanted to be an adult so badly.

Yeah! Grade one! Finally, I was going to be in a place that would actually help in my quest to obtain the knowledge I so desired. I attended a big Catholic elementary/high school combined that went from grades one through eleven. It was a bilingual school. One floor held English classes, the other French. I loved grade one—for at least two whole months. I loved learning and had some good friends. I also had a new silent crush on a boy in my class. In the 1970s most schools in Montreal adopted a system wherein classes were split into three groups: average, advanced and special needs. I learned quickly and was placed at the advanced table almost immediately. Math came to me with such ease that I questioned why I had heard people say "Girls aren't good at math." Perhaps, having heard that phrase, I was determined to prove otherwise. I was always willing to accept a challenge, and I always played to win.

Not long into grade one I asked Wanda if I could see her grade two English and math texts. I covered the material in full and told my teacher as much. Instead of praising and encouraging my progress and desire to learn, my teacher and the school's principal telephoned my parents and told them to discourage me from studying the advanced material.

I was enraged! My parents were angry! To add insult to injury, a school friend of mine had just been advanced from grade one to grade two because she, too, processed the higher level material with ease. Accordingly, I asked my parents to find out whether I could skip grade one as my friend had done. The school's answer was "No!" The principal argued that my bypassing a grade would create social hardships for both my sister and me. I confronted the principal directly. I asked him why he felt that my friend could handle the "social hardships" he had mentioned and that I could not.

He said, "Her situation is different from yours."

I asked, "How so?"

He replied, "I am not at liberty to discuss another student with you."

And that was the end of that. I later discovered that my friend's father knew the principal socially. Boy, was I pissed off!

I never understood why the school put up stop signs on my road to knowledge and freedom. At the risk of sounding like a hippie wannabe, "The system screwed me, man." Summertime was reserved for special learning projects. The summer of 1971 I convinced my mom to teach me cursive handwriting because I was fed up not knowing the adult writing code.

I coasted through grades one to three putting in as little effort as possible and always getting high grades. I reasoned that if the school would not let me skip a grade—or grades, for that matter—I would carry on teaching myself and consider my hours in school playtime. Taking control over my education was my way of asserting my freedom.

My happiest times in this first elementary school occurred during the second grade school year when my friends and I would get together and sing. Every day at lunch hour we would teach each other our favorite songs and practice singing them. We were a cute trio. We even tried to come up with some "Supremes" style dance moves. One day we decided we were ready for an audience. We stood in the middle of the playground and started to sing. Much to my surprise and joy, students of all ages, ranging from 6 to 16 years old, slowly gathered around to listen to us. And then came the applause . . .

All I remember about the applause was my response: confusion, disorientation and joy! Joy, oh joy, oh joy! I did not believe anyone would like our singing. I was thrilled! My ecstasy was short lived, however. The school principal told the crowd to disperse and then proceeded to berate us for singing "adult" songs. I argued that my parents knew I sang these songs and had no qualms about my doing so. The principal threatened to suspend me for "talking back."

I said, "Go ahead and try! It's not like I'd be missing anything anyway, so go ahead!"

He turned three shades of red, grabbed me by my arm and dragged me into his office. My two singing allies looked on in horror. I smiled back at them and said, "Don't worry. I'm not."

In his office the principal proceeded to take off his belt. I told him if he so much as touched me, I would have my parents charge him with assaulting a minor. His look of bewilderment was all I needed. I said, "Call my daddy. I'll give you his work number. Call him and see if you're allowed to hit me."

He stared at me with contempt and said, "Get out! Just get out and go back to class."

I walked out smiling, then laughing. I won! I finally won! I fought back and *won!* Joy, oh joy, oh joy.

After this incident a lot of the kids at school looked up to me, something I did not really want or expect. Later in life this fight with the principal was remembered as a sexual assault, probably because he took off his belt and I considered that sexually threatening.

My only other fond memory of grade two and this school was a boy named Charlie. Charlie started school late in the school year. I believe it was February 1972. I remember noticing him because he wore a cool black hat. Talking to him, I found out he had just moved to Montreal from Germany. I thought that was "neat." His father was in the Canadian Armed Forces and was a pilot; his family had been stationed in Germany for one year. Charlie was in grade three. He immediately confided in me that he was having problems with his math class. I offered to help him during lunch hour, since I had already finished the grade three math. When he asked me how I had done that, I told him that I had borrowed my sister's math text and had taught myself, adding that I could explain math to him by telling him the way that I had figured it out in my head.

We met at lunchtime the following day and I began tutoring him. Charlie got better and better at math and soon reached the point where he could understand it without my help. I was sad when I realized he no longer needed my assistance. I thought he would stop wanting to spend the lunch hour with me. Happily, I was wrong.

If I'm wrong and I know that I'm wrong, then I'm right that I'm wrong; so I'm right and wrong at the same time. (Janet's convoluted logic.)

Charlie and I continued to get together during lunch hour. We talked a lot about music. Both of us loved music. It was at this time that I decided I was going to be a singer lady when I grew up. Charlie asked if I would want to play an instrument too.

I answered, "My first choice is the guitar."

He asked, "Why guitar? What about piano?"

"I can't carry a piano around everywhere I go," I replied. "Besides which, I love guitar! It sounds cool. But I won't play it unless I can play it as good as a man. Do you know Glen Campbell? He can play the guitar really good. That's who I want to play like."

Charlie thought I was joking; in fact, he laughed. He said he had never heard of a girl who could play the guitar like a man. Needless to say, I was infuriated. I vowed that not only would I play the guitar like a man, but also I would play *better* than men.

Why is it that the phrase "needless to say" always prefaces something said? (Just me, meandering again.)

Charlie said, "I didn't mean to make you mad at me. I believe you can do it if you say so, man. Hell, I dare you."

And having now used the "H-E-double hockey sticks" word, I would like to remark that all of the swear words I ever wanted to know, I learned on the school bus when I was 6 years old. And I have been using them liberally ever since.

I asked Charlie which instrument he would want to play.

"Guitar and harmonica, man. Like Neil Young," he responded.

"Who's Neil Young?" I asked.

Charlie looked at me incredulously and said, "You haven't heard of Neil Young? You must know Neil Young. He's, like, the most famous Canadian musician ever!"

I insisted I did not know who Neil Young was, so Charlie asked me if I would like to have lunch at his house where he could play some records for me. I agreed with his plan, and the next day I went to Charlie's house, ready to hear some new music. We sat in his den. I remember seeing pilot memorabilia on top of the television set. Charlie was very proud that his dad was a pilot.

We were listening to records when I said, "I've heard that one." The song *Heart of Gold* was playing. "If that's Neil Young, I like him. Except he sounds like a whining cat. But it's a good song . . . if someone else would sing it. But it *is* a good song."

Charlie was somewhat miffed. He said, "When you're older, you're going to love Neil Young. I'll bet you anything."

I said, "No, Charlie. If he sounds like a whining cat now,

he'll still sound like a fucking whining cat when I'm older."

(I saw Neil Young in concert in October 1996 as I am a *huge fan* of his music and, yes, his singing. I cannot emphasize enough my love for Neil Young and have no qualms about saying that Charlie was absolutely correct.)

"Janet! Did you just say 'F-ing'?" Charlie looked so horrified that I could not help but laugh.

"Yes, Charlie, I said the 'F' word. I swear sometimes. I actually swear a lot. I like swearing. I figure if grown-ups can do it, so can I."

The next word out of Charlie's mouth was "Fuck." I think I helped to corrupt a minor. Oh well, what the . . . hey . . .

Charlie's house burned down that weekend. I heard he moved to the West Island of Montreal. It may as well have been the moon from where I lived. I was quite devastated when I found out he was gone. Eventually I forgot about him. It is funny how, when you are a kid, it is easy to forget someone. It is stranger, still, that I remember him now. I went back to having a silent crush on the boy in my class. I do not know why, but I have always felt the need to be in love, even if the love were unrequited.

I went through grade three at the same elementary school. Not much changed. I hung out with one of my two singing buddies. The other had decided to go to Protestant school because it was rumored to provide a superior education. Since I felt there were no good reasons to stay where I was, I asked my parents if I could go to a Protestant elementary school starting in grade four. They agreed.

Before moving on to discuss my Protestant school days, I should address the underlying reason that I wished to change schools, that I wanted a brand new environment. Although I had friends at school, none of them socialized with me outside of school. The older I grew, the more aware I became of this situation and its effect on me. I became more and more cynical and sad. If it were not for the summer vacations my family enjoyed, I might have fallen into a depressed state earlier in life. I am just guessing. The main thing is that I thought a change would make me feel happier.

Backtracking for a moment, I have to say that my family's

summer vacations afforded me tremendous joy. Our trip to Jamaica in 1971 was a big deal to me. We flew first class and stayed at a private villa for one week and at a well-known hotel for the remaining ten days. From the hotel we went on daily excursions around the island. I remember the vacation quite vividly. I also recall that when we returned to Montreal, a post-holiday blue funk set in. My neighborhood friends did not seem too interested in hanging out with me. I noticed a difference in their treatment of me right away. So I became a homebody starting that year and remained a homebody for a very long time afterwards. During my years of self-imposed solitude, I taught myself many hobbies: knitting, crochet, needlepoint, drawing and, of course, music. But I digress.

I am sorry. I just had to work in the phrase "But I digress." Do not ask me why. Wait! I know why. Manic people perpetually digress. It's who we are; it's what we do. (Me again.)

All right! If my neighborhood "friends" did not want to know me, it was OK. I would meet a whole slew of new kids in my new school. Fine with me. I had not given up on people just yet. I cropped my long brown hair short the summer of '73, just one week before starting grade four at the new school. It was time for changes, even if I had to make them happen myself.

Chapter 2

OK, so the changes included a cast. Just four days before school started, I fell off my white bicycle and fractured my left wrist. I was happy. I could get everyone to sign my cast. That would be cool. All of my friends had broken some bone or other, and I just wanted to be "in."

The new Protestant elementary school came with a new set of rules. In my previous school there were no dress codes or gym classes, and students could go home for lunch if they so desired. The new school insisted girls wear white blouses with blue or red tunics or pantsuits, and a school gym uniform consisting of red shorts and white T-shirts was also required. I loathed red then, now and forever! Blue, on the other hand, was and is my favorite color. Blue it was.

I bit the bullet. I thought I could tolerate these minor infringements on my personal freedom considering that I would receive a superior education and have the opportunity to make new, real friends. I was aware of the new school's rules before I made my decision to change schools. What I did not know was that the boys had no dress code.

I am a feminist, which is probably apparent by now, except that I hate the word "feminist," for it rings of feminine superiority. I am really more of an "equalist." I am fully aware I could have used the word "egalitarian"; however, egalitarian, to me, sounds like it has something to do with horses. I prefer equalist, and so what if I made it up. Someone has to come up with new words, or languages would not exist.

As an equalist I believe women and men should live by the same rules. Yes, I believe in both equal pay for equal work, and equal employment opportunities. And although I am a Catholic, I resent the patriarchal system the Church employs.

It is official. This is a diatribe—my first so far. Diatribes are très manic.

I do not believe, however, that men should cease and desist from treating women courteously. Please open the door for me and pay for dinner. Please bring me flowers or chocolates. As "the kang" said, *"Treat Me Nice."* (I fell in love with Elvis when I was 9 and he is still "the kang" to me. I eat peanut butter every day in his honor. With honey, a woman's prerogative.)

My first week at my new school in September 1973 was hellish. To my horror, I discovered immediately that I was behind in math. I caught up to my classmates in about a week and forged ahead of them within a couple of months, but the idea that I had been *behind* in something—anything—bruised my ego and instilled a vague fear of failure.

I made friends rapidly and found a new boy to love from afar. My best friend at school was a boy, and for a long time my closest friends were male.

I loved my teacher. She had beautiful handwriting and I closely copied her style. Whenever I see anything that seems right to me, I tend to take it in so it becomes part of me. Maybe copying people is my way of honoring and remembering them and the positive effects they have had on my life. Unfortunately, I have soaked up some negative ideas and traits along the way, too. Hence the depression.

I enjoyed the academic challenges presented in my new school. I still wanted to be first in everything . . . except gym. I hated gym. I will always hate gym. Gym was nonacademic and, therefore, something I could not control. I was not athletic and had no interest whatsoever in sports. The point is that I knew if I put in the effort in an academic subject, I could get an "A"; but no amount of effort would get me an "A" in gym class. Therefore, I could not control the situation. Therefore, gym sucked!

Therefore, however, hence—these words remind me that at age 9 I decided I would become a lawyer when I grew up. I figured the odds of my making a living as a singer lady were unfavorable, so I made an alternate career choice just to be safe. Also, I was a greedy and ambitious child. I often said, "A man's castle is his home," and I wanted my castle badly.

You know what? I think some part of depression is rooted in the loss of one's true self. When we are tiny tots, we know exactly what and whom we like or hate and why. We never worry or even ponder *how* we will get to where we want to be. We just assume that we can. "I think I can, I think I can," said the little engine that could. Nobody warned the engine it could run out of steam. As we grow, we compromise (the little engine is now teetering on top of the hill). Compromise leads to a lot of can'ts (the train is backing down the hill). Ultimately compromise, for some of us, breaks the spirit (and now the engine is completely derailed).

Some concessions are good. I know that. But if we spend our lives giving in to the ideals of others, we lose ourselves.

I think I done conceded one too many times. (I am thinking in a southern drawl. I often speak or think in assorted accents.)

My first concession was choosing a career outside of music. As a result, I was seldom happy in my work or in school. I guess the great depression really began when I was 9 years old, and not 10 as I had originally thought. Certainly the seeds were planted in that year, 1973. The seeds outright sprouted, grew and had little baby sprouts by the time I turned 10.

In addition to compromise, I think rules are another possible root of depression. Society has rules and laws that are good and justified. The negative rules to which I am referring are those arbitrary rules designed to achieve conformity (e.g., school dress codes). I define "conformity" as "being the same as everyone else." Why on earth would anyone want to be a conformist? We are all different from each other, thank God. I do not want to be told what or whom I should like. I do not want some fashion police dictating whether or not the miniskirts and leggings I love are *outré*. Black and blue are my favorite colors. Period.

I do believe this is diatribe number two. Whatever.

I smoke and that is that. My hair is short because I like it that way. Basically, I do what I do! But that is now. Up until now, I compromised a lot.

That same September 1973 my parents bought me a classical guitar and enrolled me in group lessons. I was the only girl in a class of about ten students, ranging from ages 6 through 10. The lessons were held on Saturday mornings in my school. At the first lesson we learned one scale, two chords and how to tune the guitar. I know this should not make me laugh, but . . . apparently the head instructor had a nervous breakdown following this first lesson and was never heard from again.

I practiced about twenty minutes a day. I remember my fingers being in extreme pain. The assistant instructor, now head instructor, encouraged me a great deal. I was able to strum The Beatles' *Eleanor Rigby* by the end of the first month. That song saddened me terribly, for I dreaded being alone like Eleanor when I grew up. And my first month was my last. I did not like giving up my Saturday morning cartoons. I guess I was not ready to commit to learning the guitar at this time. But I left the lessons knowing how to read chord diagrams, and with that knowledge in hand I reasoned I could teach myself how to play. Although I picked up my guitar from time to time over the next few years, I did not really commit to it until I was 12.

What else can I say about fourth grade? I was a voracious reader and was particularly fond of the "Nancy Drew" series by Carolyn Keene. Nancy presented a strong, intelligent female character, and I liked this strong representation of women. I loved playing jacks. Even though I was virtually a little adult by age 9, I loved my jacks. I learned this game while on vacation in Maine and brought it back with me to Montreal where seemingly no one had heard of it. Yes, I said, "in Maine." Did I go to the beach while vacationing in this Atlantic state? No, I played jacks with a boy my age at the hotel where we were both staying. Anyway, the game helped me to make friends at my new school; in fact, playing jacks became the cool thing to do. I always did my schoolwork fast and furiously so that I could have as much free time as possible. I am constantly on a mission to have free time. Sometimes I think I am lazy, but perhaps spoiled is a more accurate description. I do not know. Is it spoiled to want to do the things that give you joy? Because if that is the case, I have to think all the souls in Heaven are spoiled rotten. What do I do with my free time? Stuff, stuff and more stuff. I am never idle. I never stop thinking. Everyone tells me to relax, and my response is that I do relax; I call it "sleep."

My favorite television show in the '70s was *Get Smart*. I watched it religiously, laughing at the same jokes over and over. Sitcoms are still my favorite television fare. I mean, entertainment that gives us laughter has got to be a good thing.

At this point I would like to talk about those silent crushes to which I have alluded. I have almost always had crushes on boys or men who had no interest in me—crushes that I kept to myself; hence the word "silent." Now that I am older and wiser and medicated, I realize that I was making a habit of choosing men who were clearly out of reach and that I was forcing myself to put on an act when around them. I was hiding my true feelings and, as a result, my true self. I was pinning my happiness on whether or not I thought these men could someday be mine. My self-esteem had vanished. I went from being a confident, happy child; into a depressed, insecure teenager; and ultimately into a worried, sad, needy adult. All because I could not get a date?! I was blaming all of my problems on not having the boyfriend I wanted, when in fact I was mentally ill. Who knew?

Now that I enjoy a modicum of sanity, I know I was not really looking for a man back then. If I were, I would have chosen one who cared for me. In reality, I had no desire to give up my independence because there were too many things I wanted to do that required my being single. For example, had I married in my twenties, I would not have learned grade ten classical guitar; I would not have had the time needed to do so. It is equally doubtful that I ever would have sung and played guitar in public. I would not have written songs. I would not be writing this book . . . and on it goes.

No! My plan for me from a very early age was to stay single until I was at least 32 years old. By holding off on marriage until later in life, I would have the free time necessary to achieve my childhood ambition of becoming the world's best guitar player. Also, I would be old enough to know exactly what I was looking for in a man.

I may not be the world's best guitar player yet, but I have lots of time.

All right. I am now 36, single and still utterly clueless when it comes to men.

Chapter 3

The summer of 1974 was great! My family vacationed in Denmark for two weeks and explored this beautiful country where my dad had been born and raised. We saw the Little Mermaid statue in the harbor; we visited Tivoli Gardens, Hans Christian Andersen's house and Legoland (a child's heaven); and we ate! Denmark with its world-famous pastries was my Utopia, as my sweet tooth, like hope, springs eternal. The men were good looking, too.

When my family returned to Montreal, I was looking for something to do; so I taught myself how to type in about a week. Although I thought I would require this skill at some point in my life, learning to type was actually more of an alternate-career-type move. I wanted something to fall back on in case I did not succeed in becoming either a lawyer or a musician.

I was eagerly looking forward to my second year at the Protestant school. I could hardly wait to learn new things, and I was anxious to see my friends again. But this year was going to be different. On the first day back, I nervously walked into the school wearing a blue denim pantsuit. Immediately I was told that I was not dressed according to the code. As a little lawyer-in-training, I argued that the code required a red or blue tunic or pantsuit and that I was, in fact, wearing a blue *cotton* pantsuit. The "they"—they who be "they" and not "us" (in this case, teachers and principals)—said that the denim looked like jeans. I simply retorted that the code did not forbid the wearing of *cotton,* and I won the argument. By the second week of school there were a lot of denim pantsuits in the school's hallowed halls. Me, I was thrilled that I had finally managed to even the score. The boys had already been dressing as they saw fit, and now the girls could too. Life was sweet.

As I have already noted, I was born September 18, 1964. My birthday basically fell on a day two weeks into the start of each new school year and, as such, was seldom recognized. I was always asked "When is your birthday?" long after it had passed, and the oversight always saddened me. OK, I know I am overly sensitive about my birthday, but I feel a birthday is the one day in the year that celebrates a person's life—a person's existence—and so it should be recognized, acknowledged. I am a Virgo, which by definition is someone who constantly strives for perfection. And that is true. The other chief traits of my sign are that Virgos are nature lovers and are generally modest. Well, you cannot get me to walk on grass if there is perfectly good pavement around, I deem myself a shade bunny, and I consider dining alfresco roughing it. And I know you must be overwhelmed by my modesty now!

It's pretty difficult to write an autobiography without being self-indulgent. How many ways can one say "I"? I'm actually rather insecure, but damned if I'm going to let that stop me!

My grade five teacher was great! Her specialty was music, and I loved it when she taught the class to sing in harmony. As an alto I was relegated to singing background harmony, but my teacher recognized my love for music and chose me to play the Autoharp for the Christmas pageant. Playing the Autoharp, a stringed instrument, inspired me to try my hand at guitar once more. Slowly but surely, I learned new chords and new songs. I was happy.

In February 1975 my family moved to a new house in a new neighborhood. The house itself was beautiful and large. I finally got my very own bedroom and, as a preteen, that was important to me. I befriended a girl who lived around the block from me.

Are you hearing a "but"?

The move resulted in our being zoned out of our former school district. I could no longer go to the school I so loved. Yes, despite the dress code nonsense, I loved that school. I loved my teacher, my friends.

What can I say about the next school? I *hated* it with a passion from my first day in attendance to my last. The school was very small, very old and rife with cliques. I discovered right away that many of the students and teachers were somehow related to each other. I found this odd. Not only did I have to contend with the clannishness of the students and teachers, but also I lived in fear of the principal who carried around a baseball bat everywhere and all the time. I found the school so strange that within days I dubbed it something akin to The Asylum.

I had no friends at this school during my first half-year in attendance, February to June 1975. I did not even have my usual silent crush. The teachers seemed smug. Everyone seemed smug. The school was in an old-money neighborhood and it showed. That this school was renowned for offering the best public education in the city mattered not. I was unhappy. I was accustomed to more modern, cheerful surroundings. The Asylum was a small brown brick building that dated back to the early 1920s, and I never did care for old buildings. The plumbing in the school was ancient, the ventilation consisted of opening windows, and we students who commuted to school ate lunch in the gym, which smelled like . . . a gym.

Man, I'm whining. Ah well, I'm gonna whine some more—I mean, my diatribe continues.

The Asylum had a unique classroom structure in which two grades were combined into one classroom. For example, students in grade two could attend the grade one/two class or the grade two/three class depending upon their performance. Grade six/six was basically advanced grade six. Because we were new to the school, my sister Wanda and I were placed in grades five/six and four/five respectively without regard to our prior academic standings.

I realized instantly that grade four/five was intended for students of low to average grade five abilities. I took my complaint to my teacher, saying I belonged in grade five/six. She said I would have to discuss my situation with the principal, the guy with the bat. He argued that it was against school policy to place siblings in the same classroom. I countered that there was a set of twins in my class.

The principal stated, "Twins are exceptional."

"I'm exceptional," I retorted. "I've always gotten straight As, and I deserve to be in grade five/six. Period!"

Gripping his bat in both hands, the principal growled, "I do not care for your tone of voice, young lady. I am in charge of this school, and you will treat me with respect. Do you understand, or do I have to make myself clearer?"

"I understand," I replied, "but I don't think that my dad will. In fact, I think I'll tell my dad all about this conversation when I get home." Shaking, I left his office.

I began to cry uncontrollably, so I went to the girls' bathroom and stayed there until I could regain my composure. I was afraid of the principal. Truly afraid. And no one had ever scared me before.

Once home, I told my parents all about this confrontation. My dad took me to school the following day and discussed my class placement with the principal, alone. When my dad, smiling, left the principal's office, I knew I had gotten my way. The principal told me to go up to the grade five/six classroom and apologized for "any misunderstanding."

Wanda was thrilled to see me walk into her classroom. She was finding it difficult to make friends as well. At least now we would have each other.

Wanda and I have been called the "Bobbsey Twins" throughout our lives. We look so different from each other that people usually assume we are friends and not sisters. The "twin" moniker relates to our closeness. I have always tried to include Wanda in my activities, and she has done the same for me. Right now we share a basement apartment in our parents' house. We do have the occasional verbal altercation, but in general we get along well. I love Wanda more than she knows. She has always supported me. She has stuck by me through thick and thin, in sickness and in health. Wanda, too, suffers from mental illness; therefore, she can understand and relate to me. Her illness started later in life than did mine and consists mainly of depression and paranoia. She does not suffer from the delusions and voices and mania that I know so well. But there exists no scale on which to rate the level of one's suffering.

Prozac, Zoloft, Ativan, Haldol—I'll bet you've heard these drug names before and that's sad. Mental illness has reached such epic proportions that it's now trendy to be on "meds" (the shorter and more hip word for "medications"). Hell, I'm so "in," I'm too "in."

I was a lot happier in my new grade five/six classroom, or should I say, I was a lot less depressed. The new classroom, located on the second (top) floor, had many windows and was much more cheerful than my previous classroom had been. The teacher was somewhat harsh, but her attitude did not really bother me because I was in grade five/six and that was what I wanted.

Essentially, grade five/six was grade six. We studied sixth grade English, French, math and history. In math I excelled. The students in this class were very competitive, and I relished the challenge they presented me. This was the first time I vied with people on my level. I remember well the math duel that involved me and a boy named Steve. Steve was nice, and he and I got along great; but we each wanted to best the other in math. I remember my first 100%. It was fantastic, glorious . . . until I realized the only place to go from there was down. So I worked especially hard to maintain 100%s and managed a streak of ten in a row. Then came a heartbreaking 98%. I was so embarrassed. My classmates mocked my 98% saying that I was "not all that smart." Insulting my intelligence was the most hurtful thing a person could do to me when I was 10 years old because my academic prowess was the only thing over which I felt I had control. Grades, test scores, meant everything to me.

My duel partner Steve was a nice, cute, popular boy. I was at the age where the body stores fat for impending adolescence. My hair was long and straggly, and I felt I was sorely lacking in the looks department. But Steve always made me feel beautiful. He liked me despite the pressures placed upon him by his friends. He included me, and I remember him now for his gallantry.

I did not have a crush on Steve. I was in the habit of reserving my crushes for those out of reach. It was a bad habit. I had no inkling of just how bad it was.

Chapter 4

The Wizard of Oz.
I hate what *The Wizard of Oz* represents to me. With reason.
At the end of January 1975 the school decided to put on the play *The Wizard of Oz*. Having arrived at the school after the major casting had been completed, I was eligible only for the role of jitterbug. I accepted the part because the play's rehearsals were held during English period, and I would have done just about anything to avoid my English class. All classes wherein grading was subjective made me nervous. Wanda, too, played a jitterbug. The role consisted of dancing. That was it. Just a frenzied dance similar to a square dance.
TRAUMA TIME:
In 1990 I remembered witnessing a murder. Was it real? Was it a vivid recollection of a nightmare? I don't really know. I believe it did happen, and so I shall describe the murder in detail. But you, the reader, must understand that this recount may be nothing more than a lifelike delusion—a delusion that culminated in my becoming paranoid.
It was May 23, 1975. We students had been rehearsing *"Oz"* since February and were now doing the final dress rehearsals. Out of the blue, a classmate, Karen, asked me if I would like to play baseball after school. Never having been included in any out-of-school activities

with the kids from The Asylum, I was eager for the chance to socialize with them, to get to know them. The only thing I ever really wanted out of school, besides knowledge, was to make friends. I called my mom to ask for permission to play. She asked me where I would be playing and how I would get home. I told her that I was going to the park located behind my previous school and that I would take a city bus home before dark. She said OK.

Throughout my childhood I always made sure my parents knew where I was. I had heard too many news reports about missing children, rape and murder; and I took these reports to heart. I never stayed out after dark. I was afraid to do so. I deemed myself extremely fortunate that I had a stay-at-home mom. Knowing she was home made me feel safe, happy and loved—as happy as I could feel.

I could not wait for school to let out that day. Finally! The last class ended and I went with Karen to her house. She wanted to bring her books home and to change into blue jeans. The baseball game was set to begin at 4:00 p.m., so we had about a half-hour to get to the park.

While Karen changed, I waited in the living room with her older brother Dan. Dan was in grade six/six at The Asylum. I did not really know him, but I knew I found him strange. He stared at me a lot; his vacant gaze unnerved me.

Dan was lying on the couch in his pajamas. Ostensibly he had been home nursing a flu that day. He offered me some orange juice, which I declined. I was still waiting for Karen to come back downstairs when I heard a knock at the front door. Dan, too sick or too lazy to get up, asked me to get the door. I opened the door, and to my total astonishment I recognized the older of the two girls at the door from my Girl Guide days.

As a young child I had joined Brownies because it was the trendy thing to do in my neighborhood. I went on to Girl Guides for about a month. I think I joined Guides because I loved the royal blue uniform they sported. For sure, it was not because I wanted to go camping! You cannot pay me to camp. Girl Guides did teach me one important lesson: Be prepared. And I am. I always have a pack of matches on me in case my lighter runs out of fluid.

Jane, the older girl whom I knew from Guides, was truly surprised to see me. At least six months had passed since I had left Girl Guides. Jane accompanied a little girl from The Asylum named Sherry whom I recognized immediately. In fact, I was relieved to see Sherry for reasons I knew not. Jane informed me that she was baby-sitting Sherry. And I then discovered that Jane would be playing baseball with us.

At long last, Karen came downstairs, ready to go. The four of us began the walk to the park located about 15 minutes away on foot from Karen's house. As we were walking, I happened to look back where I saw Dan, now dressed, following us with a baseball bat in hand. Again I was unnerved. He *was* supposed to be sick, after all.

We arrived at the park at 4:00 p.m., just as the other players were showing up. The majority were kids from The Asylum; but some were kids from my previous school, my happy school, and I was glad to see their familiar faces.

Once Dan arrived with the only bat, the game commenced. Although I never particularly cared for sports, I found myself enjoying baseball. I really liked being the batter, probably because I managed to hit the ball, and I just found it fun to be with the other kids. I played left field when not batting. I could not catch the ball to save my life. So, based on my observance of the game, left field seemed the right place for a player of my caliber. In other words, the ball seldom flew in that direction.

I was having a super time when I noticed it was becoming dark. Quickly, I made my apologies to the other kids and told them that I had to leave right away. The kids tried to convince me to stay and finish the game, but I said I could not. Sherry, who had been flying a kite while the rest of us played baseball, looked somewhat sad when she saw I was leaving. I asked Jane, the baby-sitter, how much longer she was supposed to watch Sherry.

Jane replied, "Just until her dad gets home from work."

"And when is that?" I asked.

"Around six o'clock. Why?" Jane was looking rather miffed.

"I think Sherry looks tired." And turning my attention towards Sherry, I asked the little girl where she lived.

"Just a block from here," Sherry replied, pointing in the direction of her house.

Looking at my watch, I said to Jane, "It's just about six o'clock now. Why don't I walk Sherry home so you can finish the game? It's not a problem for me."

Jane responded, "No, that's not a good idea. I've been baby-sitting Sherry for a month, and her dad is supposed to pay me today."

"But Sherry wants to go home *now*, Jane. She's tired. I'll walk her home, and you can go pick up your money when you're ready."

Jane, very angry now, said, "No! It's none of your business what I do with her. Her dad left me in charge of her, not you!"

And so I told Sherry that Jane would not let me take her home and that I had to leave right away. By now it was almost completely dark outside; so I felt it urgent that I get home or, in the very least, that I get to the bus stop. I rapidly walked away from the park. And then my shoelace came undone. Damned shoelaces!

Tall hedges surrounded the area of the park where we had been playing. I was well beyond these hedges and out of sight of the players when the lace came undone. Stopping to retie my shoelace, I saw Sherry's kite falling to the ground in my direction. I decided to retrieve the kite for her. And I was just behind the hedges when I saw The Thing.

I do not know why, but I remember that for a long time I mentally referred to the forthcoming incident as The Thing and was perpetually frightened that someone would discover I knew all about The Thing.

So here is The Thing: peeking through the hedges, I saw three of the kids bludgeon Sherry to death with a baseball bat. The three were Jane, Dan and Scott. The latter two attended school with me at The Asylum. I do not know which school Jane attended.

I thought I was seeing things. There was no way they could be hitting Sherry. I decided to try to get a closer look. Crawling behind the hedges, I managed to get within 15 feet of the attack site. To my horror and eternal sorrow, I saw Sherry's lifeless body lying in the grass. She was covered in blood.

The three who had murdered her were laughing and disputing who had won the game.

I was trying to understand: What "game" were they talking about?

And then Dan said, "The winner is the one who splits her head open first. I won."

That was enough. I crawled, crouched, stood up and ran away from the park as fast as I could. I wrote a song called *Running* in 1990, just prior to recalling The Thing.

Running

I tried to deny
Yeah, I wanted to hide
Running away from the rules that have beaten me down
Running ahead 'cause I won't let them pull me around
Stop, catch a breath, and they'll push you right into the
ground.

Sometimes, I used to pretend
But now it's too hard to bend
Bend and they'll break you and capture you under their spell
Bend and they'll pull you down into their own living hell
Stop, catch a breath, and you'll find that it all rings a bell.

Oh, I walked fast and I found my way home
Yeah, I walked home and I found it's my way.

I covered my eyes
'Cause I don't want to despise
Quick, steal a glimpse, and the goodness is all that you see
Turn, look again, and the spell breaks and sets your soul free
Stop, catch a breath, and I wonder why it's up to me.

Chapter 5

I took a full week of sick days following Sherry's murder. My mom could not understand my wanting to stay home because she knew that I had always prided myself on never missing school.

I did not tell my mom about Sherry. I did not tell anyone about Sherry. I kept the murder to myself because I had a very real fear that anyone who knew about Sherry would be murdered too. I remember asking Wanda if Sherry had been in school during the week in which I had stayed at home. Wanda informed me that she had not seen the little girl. Even though I *always* confided in Wanda, I did not and could not tell her about the murder I had witnessed. I was hoping for a miracle. I was desperately hoping that Sherry was alive and that I had imagined the murder.

As I have already noted, the murder and its aftermath may be delusions. What troubles me, though, is that I have all these details— facts and feelings—that I recall now as clearly as I recall my first cigarette (which was immediately followed by my second cigarette).

I was terrified to go back to school. I devised a plan: I would pretend nothing had happened, I would be especially friendly with the kids who had been at the baseball game that day, and, above all, I would be *cheerful*.

My plan . . .

You know the old adage about telling lies? If you tell one lie, then you may have to lie to cover up the first lie, and so on? I dug my own grave that first day back at The Asylum. Since no one attempted to hurt, maim or kill me, I determined that my plan, such as it was, was working. I put on my "mask of steel" that day and wore it faithfully until my Big Breakdown in 1993.

I thought a mask of steel
Concealed the love and pain I feel
Guess I was only fooling me.

Excerpt from song "Mask of Steel" © *1990, J. M. Knudsen*

I still pull out my mask and dust it off occasionally. Indeed, I believe that most mentally ill people have their masks. Hell, everyone puts on a face now and then. Shakespeare's famous line "All the world's a stage" echoed in my mind continuously during my first and subsequent breakdowns. After a while, I truly doubted that anyone was real. I mean, if people appeared happy, I thought they must be faking it; if they appeared sad, I thought they were looking for sympathy. Either way, I did not believe they were being real.

So May 23, 1975, is the official start date of my great depression and paranoia and mania . . .

I pepper my writing with ellipses—or dot-dot-dots, as I call them—because that is how my thinking operates, often incomplete or open ended. My mind is always forging ahead to the next topic. Being manic is like being in a race without a finish line in sight, ever.

Doctors tell me that I have a chemical imbalance, and they are correct. The meds I take do work. They sedate me and quell my delusions for the most part, and sedating me is rather like trying to sedate an elephant with an Aspirin. But thankfully, the meds came in and the mask came off . . . slowly. I must state, however, that I believe the trauma of Sherry's murder, whether the murder was real or imagined, was a factor in my illness. In fact, I know it. It was not until I remembered Sherry's death that the floodgates of depression and despair opened uncontrollably, with paranoia and delusions soon to follow. And it was not until my psychiatrist determined the correct combination of drugs that I was able to talk about Sherry to anyone, including me.

In school again, I smiled so much that I began to *believe* I was happy. I really thought I could forgive and forget. I kept thinking, "I just have to pretend a little bit longer. I just have to hang on until June when school lets out. I'm lucky I don't live near any of the kids from the baseball game. Thank God for that!"

Even with all my smiling, three boys from the baseball game seemed to know my secret. They were always fishing, waiting for me to slip up. One of the boys smiled the same fake smile that I wore daily, eerily mirroring and mocking me and my pain. Another repeatedly asked whether I had played baseball recently. And the third, the meanest SOB I have ever had the displeasure of meeting, kept asking me if I had seen Sherry lately.

I must apologize for using the term "SOB." I've never understood why there exists a swear that indirectly insults a person by insulting the person's mother. Perhaps I should have said "the meanest asshole . . . ." Please indulge me. I was just thinking out loud. I do that a lot.

The official story regarding Sherry's disappearance was that she was missing. The reason I hate *The Wizard of Oz* is that the kids from the murder claimed to have been rehearsing this play at the time of Sherry's disappearance. As I have already noted, it was an "incestuous" little school in that many of the students were somehow related to the teachers and to each other. It is not surprising, then, that the teachers backed up the rehearsal alibi. Everyone from the school's neighborhood backed up the rehearsal alibi. I quickly realized that even if I told the truth and talked to the police, no one would support my version of what had happened to Sherry. I would be labeled "crazy," and at age 10 the idea that I could be committed to a mental institution posed both a very real and a very frightening threat. I told no one. I cried alone.

I live in black. Black slowly and steadily worked its way into my life. First there were black shoes, then black jeans. By the time I was 24 years old, I wore black on black on black. Over the years, whenever someone would ask "Why all the black?" I perpetually replied that I was "in mourning for my lost childhood."

The thing that haunted me about my response to the black question is that I had no idea I meant it literally. I thought I was being glib. By repressing my response to Sherry's murder—always pretending it never happened, always wearing a mask of happiness—I eventually blanked the trauma out of my mind completely. I effectively erased the murder and everyone associated with it from my memory. What triggered the recall comes later.

There was one happy moment after the murder that deserves attention. In June on the last day of school, a couple of boys from my class brought in their guitars. After much persuasion (I was terrified to play in front of an audience), I played and sang a couple of songs and was applauded for my efforts. Later, one of the boys sang a song that I had never heard before, a song that I loved instantly. I learned that it was a Bob Dylan song entitled *You Ain't Goin' Nowhere.* Many years elapsed before I heard that song again. In the interim, I forgot the song completely.

I survived the remainder of the school year and had a nice summer. In July my family went on a holiday in the Laurentian Mountains located just north of Montreal. I know I needed the diversion from my thoughts. After the murder, I began to *think* constantly. I worried about everything and anything. To myself I was habitually saying, "Let me think. I need to think." I became obsessed with writing lists because I was afraid of forgetting something, anything. I no longer trusted myself to remember things. Even the pettiest item was of major consequence to me. Lists helped me to feel like I was in control, and I needed to be in control. Always in control.

My sixth grade school year proved uneventful. Most of the kids involved in the murder had moved on to high school. I was especially relieved to see that the three who had taunted me about Sherry's murder were gone. With them, the likelihood of anyone guessing my secret of having witnessed Sherry's murder was gone, too. I did not have to put on a face as much that year. Ironically, the braces I now sported on my teeth gave me a much needed excuse not to smile or laugh too much. Perhaps this was why I was so adamant about getting braces. I never really thought about it until now.

In grade six I finally found a real friend, Sarah. I often ate lunch at her house. Being able to leave the school, even if only for an hour a day, certainly improved my spirits. Sarah and I also frequented a neighborhood candy store during lunch hour. I was still enough of a child that a bag of candy was fun.

I started drinking coffee that year. One innocent mug in 1975 became ten mugs a day by the time I was 18. And I drink very strong coffee, as Europeans are wont to do. I also went on my first diet at this time. I was a bit chubby at age 11, and all of a sudden it became important to me to be thin. I weighed 110 lbs at 5'3" when I was 11; I weighed 115 lbs at 5'8" when I was 14. My weight seldom exceeded 120 lbs until I started taking meds. My thinking was definitely anorexic. Fortunately, my sweet tooth prevented me from starving myself to death. Living on a peanut butter sandwich, a chocolate bar and ten cups of coffee a day until I was 30 years old may seem rigid, but I needed the control. Weight I could control. I often referred to the word "diet" as " 'die' with a 't.' " It was a morose way of thinking, I know, but maybe my black thoughts were my brain's way of telling me to remember Sherry. Maybe.

Anyway, grade six went by rapidly and I was finally free of The Asylum and everyone associated with it. Oh, happy day.

I never saw my one friend from that school again. Sarah disappeared from my life. I began a cycle of rapidly making and losing friends that existed for many years to follow. Some might say that I had "a fear of intimacy based on my strong distrust of people and rooted in my response to the childhood trauma I endured." All I know is I would make a friend, I would lose a friend. Sometimes I pushed them away; more often they left. Either way, I was alone again. Perhaps they left because of my mental illness. It is difficult to socialize with someone who is constantly depressed. If you are happy, a depressed person can certainly bring you down over time. And many people are afraid of mania. I know that. I understand, and it is OK. Being alone I accomplished many tasks, and I achieved almost all of my personal goals. Solitude agreed with me, and I still choose to spend most of my time pursuing solitary endeavors. But I deem myself lucky that I do have some friends now—now that I have learned to stop pushing them away. It is, however, noteworthy that my closest friends suffer from mental illness too. That mentally ill people tend to turn to each other for friendship and support is a fact; indeed, it is the norm.

My family vacationed for two weeks in Prince Edward Island the summer of 1976, the summer I kissed The Asylum goodbye. (I never did go back to that school or its neighborhood. The school is now demolished, I am told.) I recall the beauty and serenity of the ocean in PEI. I remember the joy I felt when visiting the "Anne of Green Gables" house, as I loved those stories by Lucy Maud Montgomery. I was thrilled when I went on my first trail ride. All in all, I had fun! The trauma of Sherry's murder was dead and buried in my subconscious by the time I returned home to Montreal. I do not know how or why, but everything and everyone from The Asylum and the murder were now history. Forgotten.

Chapter 6

The best thing about the summer of 1976 was that I made friends in my new neighborhood. My best friend Meg and I had a lot in common. We were both high achievers who read a lot and played guitar. In the nearby undeveloped fields, we spent many sunny afternoons building multi-level tree houses and playing at being "Robin Hood" with our handmade bows and arrows. We discovered an abandoned stone house that had been gutted by fire. The house, which must have dated back to the 1800s, had a ghostly aura; but it was more interesting than it was creepy. I think I remember this summer because it was the last summer in which I played as a child would play. The following summer I was far too grown up for tree houses and role-playing games.

Meg was always telling me, "Don't sweat the little things," and "Keep the faith." I wonder if she would be surprised to know that I still regularly repeat these two phrases to myself. Indeed, these two innocent phrases often have helped me to keep going, even at my lowest moments. I suppose Meg knew that I was extremely tense and nervous back in the days when she and I were close, even if I did not.

Lise was my other good friend. She taught me the basics of piano playing and how to read music that same summer. Lise was very much into clothes and makeup and fashion in general. I guess I found my own style after knowing her. In the very least, I began to care about my appearance, my look. In the long run my love of fashion became so intense that I began to create my own clothing. I was forever drawing fashion designs in the margins of my notebooks while in high school. Miniskirts and bellbottom jeans were my thing long before they came back into fashion. Right now I am wearing a sleeveless, knit mini-dress that I designed and knitted myself. I cannot sew on a sewing machine, so all of my designs are knits.

Still on a tangent . . .

Did I say "I cannot sew"? What I meant to say is that I choose not to sew. My not sewing is one of my minor rebellions. Being an equalist, I determined long ago that I would never cook and never sew. The way I saw it, if I knew how to cook and sew, some man would one day expect me to perform these tiresome tasks for him. I do realize that many people in this world love cooking and sewing and are still equalists. I am simply not one of them.

All right. Lately I've been reconsidering my stance on sewing. Knitting is limiting my ability to design; there are only so many things one can do with wool. I hand knit. No knitting machines for me. The act of knitting is extremely meditative and relaxing, but I need a new challenge. Sewing would definitely provide that. As a manic, I always need to be learning or doing something new. That's part of the good mania, and there is such a thing as "good" mania.

The one other memorable event of the summer of '76 was that I had my first real kiss with the boy who was my latest silent crush. My friends and I were playing "truth or dare," and I happily took a dare so I could kiss this boy. Meg, Lise and I all liked him, and why not? He was older, 14 to be exact, and he was gorgeous. Unfortunately, he freaked out when I told him that I was only 11 years old, going on 12 in a couple of weeks. He did not want to know me after this admission. Whatever.

In Montreal when I was growing up, high schools encompassed grades seven through eleven. I believe the system remains the same to this day. I was overjoyed when I started grade seven. High school offered a whole new world complete with many new faces. It also offered a taste of freedom in that students in the seventh grade were permitted one elective class. My neighborhood friends and I worked out our schedules so that we would be in the same classes together as much as possible. I was reasonably happy, but tense—always on edge.

You will not believe who sat next to me in homeroom on the first day of school: Jane. Baseball, baby-sitting, bludgeoning, bloody Jane. And I had no inkling who she was. I began talking to her by introducing myself. She did not blink. She went along with the "I have never met you before" scenario. This scene presaged all of my future meetings with the lethal kids. Whenever I bumped into those kids from the baseball game/murder scene, I did not recognize them. I truly believed I was meeting them for the first time. Self-preservation? I do not know.

And now I will introduce the source of the paranoia and delusions that have plagued me since 1989: The Game. In a nutshell The Game, as I have dubbed it, is a live, unending mind game. Its players—whom I refer to as "they," "them" or "the players"—are the kids who were involved in Sherry's murder, the adults who helped in the cover-up, and the families and friends of these two groups. The players number around one hundred. That is my best estimate.

Is The Game real? In 1990 one of its players confessed to me that I was indeed the target of a game that had commenced in '89. The "Confessor," as I call him, did not elaborate on what this game was or its purpose. He merely informed me that a live mind game existed and that I was winning. More accurately, the players who were betting on me were winning.

So I know The Game was real as of 1989. I cannot state with absolute certainty that The Game started immediately following Sherry's death, nor do I know whether it has ended. My belief is that The Game did start in 1975 and is ongoing.

Whether real or imagined, The Game played a major role in my breakdown. It drove me insane, and God brought me back again. God . . . and my psychiatrist . . . and my meds.

Can you imagine just how confusing it is to have paranoia that is partly rooted in reality? The lines between reality and imagination blur. For my sanity's sake, I want to believe that the murder was a very real nightmare. But still, I cannot dismiss that there was a game . . .

I am armed with the knowledge of what went on in my mind while my tenuous hold on sanity was slipping away. The Game planted the seeds of paranoia that grew and grew until I believed the whole world was playing The Game, the whole world was evil.

It occurs to me that maybe I have had a happy, uneventful life and that my brain concocted a murder and ensuing mind game because I was bored. But the Confessor is real. Where does this knowledge leave me? I do not know.

I was generally happy in seventh grade. I had a wonderful math teacher who encouraged me to study at my own pace. He gave me the eighth grade math text and found me a private study room wherein I could teach myself. I was required to be in his classroom only to take the regular grade seven math tests. My friend Meg, who was also advanced in math, studied with me for a while; but we spent more time talking than learning. After a couple of months Meg opted to slow down a bit. She missed being in the regular classroom with the rest of the kids, I guess. Me, I carried on teaching myself and finished the grade eight math text well before the grade seven school year ended. I always wanted to be one step ahead of everyone. Still do. My song *Running* emphasizes this need.

I studied piano seriously during the 1976-77 school year. I went to a professional piano teacher, as Lise had taught me all that she could. Under the guidance of my new teacher, I went from grade three to grade five piano in one year and played Beethoven's *Moonlight Sonata* in a shopping mall as part of a year-end recital. Yeah, I did the mall scene well before it was hip. From piano I learned to read music and to appreciate classical music. I also learned that I wanted to play guitar more than ever!

My parents supported my decision to quit piano. They knew my first love was and is the guitar. So I started to teach myself guitar in earnest. I bought guitar songbooks and practiced learning by ear off of my many Rolling Stones albums.

Keith Richards. My inspiration. He is the rhythm/lead guitar player for The Rolling Stones, and he holds the esteemed position of being my all-time favorite guitar player. Hanging on my bedroom wall is a drawing I made of Keith in which he is wearing a bandanna, his eyes are closed and he has a cigarette dangling between his lips. He inspired me to play the guitar in two ways: the first is that he plays with both passion and a definitive style that made me want to recreate and build upon that sound; the second is a statement that he is reputed to have made to the effect that no woman could play the guitar as well as a man.

Considering I was and am an equalist, Keith's statement regarding women and the guitar should have riled me no end. But it did not. At the time he made that statement, I had to agree with him. I, too, had not heard a female guitar player who measured up to the men. I was not yet familiar with Bonnie Raitt or Chrissie Hynde. Happily, I can now say that I, along with many other female guitar players, do measure up. I *can* play "like a man," and I thank Keith Richards for challenging me to do so.

Tangent time. My favorite Stones song is "You Got the Silver" (Keith sings it). My thrill of a lifetime was seeing The Rolling Stones in concert, twice. (The first time I saw them live, I thought, "OK. If I were to die right now, I'd die happy.") My biggest fantasy is to someday play guitar with Keith. It could happen!

Alone in my bedroom, I spent many hours learning the guitar and practicing singing. Because I am an alto, singing presented the bigger challenge for me. I tried unsuccessfully to raise my vocal range. Ultimately, I reasoned that if I could not hit the higher notes, I would teach myself to sing lower and lower and expand my range in that direction.

I was never so insulted in all my life as when Meg told me that I had a nice voice but that I was off key, a little bit flat. I went home and made a tape of my singing that same day. Much to my chagrin, Meg was right. So I began to practice singing by taping myself and by working on the areas that needed fixing. I now sing on key, most of the time, and people tell me that I do Patsy Cline and Janis Joplin proud.

You would think a pessimist—and I was a complete pessimist after Sherry's murder—would take the easy way out. But I have always responded to challenges that I felt might have some import in my life.

I have always fought the good fight. I believe my dad deserves most of the credit for instilling some optimism in me way back when. He is the eternal optimist; he never gives up. And neither do I. Thank you, Dad.

Chapter 7

Have you ever wondered which came first, the pessimism or the depression? I will grant you that I was a cynical child—I prefer the term "mini-adult"—but pessimistic?

Earlier I stated my views on conformity, concessions and rules. Now I will add cynicism and pessimism to my list of ingredients of depression. Cynicism and pessimism are direct results of the conformity, concessions and rules forced upon us from the moment we are born (i.e., you are too young/old to . . . , or girls/boys do not . . . , or it is not polite to . . . , and so on).

First I became cynical, and cynicism begat pessimism, and pessimism begat depression, and depression begat *despair*. I would say that out-and-out despair did not figure into my life until I was in my thirties; but I did live with depression, on and off, from age 10 onward. Despair, sadly, often leads to suicide. Were it not for my strong faith in God, I would be a memory.

I know exactly when I became cynical. When I was in grade one doing grade two work and I found out that I could not skip a grade—man, I was cynical. Discovering for the first time and at such a young age that hard work does not necessarily pay off, I became *cynical*. Finding out over and over and over again that life and people are not always fair led to *pessimism*. **Believing** that people and life are not fair, I fell into *depression*. Finally, the realization that nobody really gives a damn whether or not *I* find life fair resulted in *despair.*

In writing this book, I am trying to overcome some of my own despair. In my 1990 song *Mask of Steel* from which I have already quoted, I write:

> *I sit here wondering 'bout you*
> *And I worry 'bout you, too*
> *But I have to go away*
> *Lost in buried sorrows*
> *Still bleeding in my soul, so*
> *Can I please have another day.*

Excerpt from song "Mask of Steel" © 1990, J. M. Knudsen

These days I am a lot happier than I am sad. I am definitely optimistic. But still some days I cry, seemingly for no reason, and it takes every fiber of my being to stop the tears. The depression part of manic depression really, really sucks!

Sometimes the physical release of crying is all that I need to feel better. But I often try to laugh my tears away. I consider tears futile in that they cannot effect change, so I laugh them away when I can.

There is one other item that I wish to discuss regarding depression. I think impatience is the water that helps depression grow and flourish in your heart, mind and soul. I hope the following poem of mine helps to open your heart to the possibility of happiness.

Patience

PATIENCE
I cannot negotiate time
To suit my needs and wants and desires
PATIENCE
I cannot turn back the clock
To correct my mistakes
      BESIDES
God tells me patience is all you need
PATIENCE IS THE SEED OF THE TREE OF FAITH

Poem "Patience" © 1995, J. M. Knudsen

This chapter is purposely short. A person suffering from depression would find reading this chapter daunting, if not overwhelming.

Chapter 8

I was a pessimist the summer of 1977. I used to argue that pessimism was logical. A pessimist typically expects the worst to happen and, if proven right, will not suffer too much disappointment. If a pessimist is wrong and something good happens, then the positive outcome seems especially sweet.

I am now an optimist. As I grew older, it occurred to me that anticipating the worst was an open invitation for the worst to come into my life.

Like, I'm attracting negative vibes into my space, man. (Valley girl accent in my head.)

But I really do believe in the power of thought. One sad person in a roomful of people can bring down everyone present. I know. I recently went to see my psychiatrist on the psych ward—I was having my first manic-depressive breakdown in over five years—and I had to wait on the ward for over an hour to see him. In that short space of time, I became first edgy and then physically drained. I could not wait to leave. I pleaded with my doctor to treat me as an outpatient because I felt a stay on the psych ward would prove detrimental, if anything. (I am well, now.)

My family vacationed in Massachusetts the summer of 1977. The vacation was OK. My spirits were low, and I do not think anything would have cheered me up at that time. We stayed at a cottage near the beach but, to me, the beach was boring. I did not believe in tanning, and since the Atlantic Ocean is extremely cold at any time of year, swimming was out. In addition, I could not relax. I have never mastered the art of doing nothing. In fact, I remember my friend Lise's mother telling me that the only time she had ever seen my face at peace was when I was sleeping.

I've heard many self-help gurus condone and encourage the art of meditation and relaxation. When I was on the psych ward, my doctor signed me up for a meditation workshop. Did I relax at this workshop? God, no. I told the leader of the group that I could not possibly relax if I wasn't allowed to smoke. At least when I was younger, I could sleep through the night. Now, I wake up around 2:00 a.m. every night—to smoke. Oh, what a bitter irony . . .

Like all preteens, I used to host and attend slumber parties. After one such party Meg informed me that I talked in my sleep. I have no idea what I said while sleeping. All I know is that my friends would look at me strangely in the mornings. I still talk in my sleep. I guess it *is* hard to get me to shut up.

Another bad habit, one that I developed during a stay on the psych ward, is midnight snacking. Oh well. To sum up my sleep disorders: I talk in my sleep, I eat in my sleep, and I smoke in my sleep. And I am currently as relaxed as I have ever been!

Summer ended all too soon, and it was time to go back to school. Grade eight was much like grade seven had been. I had my same group of friends, and I continued to study advanced everything. On the bright side, Bloody Jane moved away a few months into the school year. And it was at this time that a new expression came into my life that I hung onto for many years to follow: "I'm bored."

"How are you, Janet?" they would ask.

"I'm bored," I would reply.

"How can you possibly be bored?" Them again.

*"How can you **not** be bored?" Me.*

I do not know how many times I had this same conversation . . . with "them." The them who be "they." The they who had played baseball and who now played the ensuing mind game. In grade eight I noticed there were a lot of new faces, faces I thought I had not seen before—faces from the murder and The Asylum. The they who be "they." Once again they were fishing to see if I knew anything about Sherry's murder. The "I'm bored" response really pissed them off. I simply did not recognize the "they."

Before I continue, I need to clarify that although I did not consciously recognize the kids associated with Sherry's murder, I did treat them quite differently from the way that I treated my other, real friends. I now realize that subconsciously I must have known exactly who "they" were and that my responses to them were careful, guarded and often entirely dishonest. I lied. I lied and I lied. Every time I talked to them, I lied. Away from them, I would find myself wondering *why* I had so brazenly prevaricated. Indeed, I thought there must be something seriously wrong with me, and I felt terrible guilt over the whole lying thing. I now figure that the lies were a form of self-preservation.

The Game, as I now see it, consisted of eight major components all with which I am well acquainted: the "I don't know you" game, repetitious questions, mimicry, mirroring, following/stalking, eavesdropping, the "friend/not friend" game and the fact that The Game never ends. I must reiterate that I was not onto the mind game until the advent of the Confessor in 1990.

The "I don't know you" game began when the players discerned that I did not recognize Bloody Jane. Players would approach me carefully in an attempt to determine whether or not I recognized them. Once they realized that I did not in fact remember them, they would comport themselves as though we were meeting for the very first time. Whenever two or more years had elapsed in which I did not see certain players, these same players would enact this same charade again. I was constantly meeting everyone for the first time. As of 1989 the players are aware that I no longer forget them, regardless of how much time passes between meetings.

Repetitious questions were another component of The Game. I do not know how many times I have been asked the following same five questions since Sherry's murder. Worse, I do not know why I did not *notice* the repetitions. Not only would different players ask me these same five questions, but also a single player would go through the motions of these questions again and again. So it must have irked the players that my responses to their interrogations were utterly inconsistent. I am aware that these questions are commonplace, seemingly innocent questions that we have all heard before. However, when the same person asks you the same questions over and over again, the pattern forms a mind game. The questions and some of my responses are as follows:

Q: "What's your favorite color?"
A: "Blue." Alternately, "Black."

Q: "Do you have the time?"
A: "I never wear a watch." Alternately, "My watch says . . ."

Q: "Do you consider yourself normal?" (Why would anyone ask this?)
A: "Yes, I'm normal." Alternately, "I'm 'A-B-normal.'" (The "A-B-normal" response often procured confused looks. I explained that it would be normal to say "abnormal," whereas to say "A-B-normal" truly is abnormal. Somehow, I do not think they understood me.)

Q: "If you could have power, money or fame, which would you choose?"
A: "Power." Alternately, "money" or "fame." (I was extremely inconsistent in my responses to this question. For the record, my real and logical response would have to be money from which one can derive fame and power. But I do not care about material things. I have a car and a guitar and those are the only material things I truly desire. To me, everything else is bonus.)

Q: "Can I bum a smoke?"
A: "Yes." Alternately, "Do you smoke? Because if you do, you'd better figure out a way to buy your own cigarettes. I have my own habit to support."

And so ends the five questions aspect of The Game.

Another part of The Game was mimicry. The players would try to copy the tone of my voice, the way I laughed and the expressions I commonly used. If I said, for example, that I was "peachy," all of the players became peachy when asked.

Mirroring was similar to mimicry except that it was more visual. The players would mirror my facial expressions, my body language, my clothing, the way I walked, the way I held a cigarette . . . and on it goes.

The fifth element, following/stalking, represented The Game at its most extreme level. The same groups of people followed me from school to school, from bar to bar, from city to city—even going so far as to follow me out of the country. What perturbs me most about this aspect of The Game is that the players moved en masse. The same subgroups of people seemed to stick together forever.

Next was eavesdropping, which I know is not entirely a delusion of mine because I caught some of the players red-handed. They were standing at the door to my apartment, listening. I saw them through the peephole; I heard them running through the halls. The players used eavesdropping to drive me over the edge. I would say something in my apartment, only to hear it reiterated, sometimes verbatim, later that same day. At the time, I honestly began to believe that I must be very psychic, at least up until I caught the players at my door.

The seventh element of The Game was the "friend/not friend" ploy. At first meeting, players would be extremely friendly towards me by inviting me out, by phoning me and by introducing me to their other friends. And these friendships would last just long enough so that I would be truly hurt when the players decided that the time was right to freeze me out of their circles. This element of The Game was especially cruel because there were always other new players who would come forward and repeat the cycle. Over time, I became completely disenchanted with the idea of having or making friends. It now takes a very long time for me to establish a friendship, for me to trust someone.

The final element of The Game was simple: The Game never

ends.

OK, that was the mind game in a nutshell. Can I prove The Game was real? Is real? The answer is "No." However, my description of The Game is accurate, my paranoia certainly was born of this game, and I will refer back to The Game throughout my story.

Chapter 9

I win!

As grade eight was drawing to an end, the time came for us students to choose our classes for the following school year. My schedule would not work out were I to study advanced grade nine English; however, there would be no scheduling conflicts whatsoever were I to be promoted to the tenth grade. Since I had been studying advanced everything anyway, my guidance counselor asked me how I would feel about bypassing grade nine entirely and going directly into grade ten.

How would I feel?!

I told my counselor that I would be very happy to skip grade nine. Very happy! (It was a long time coming, I know, but I *finally* got my own way.)

The counselor clarified that I would require both my parents' permission and the principal's consent in order to skip the grade but that he felt certain my bypassing grade nine was the best possible course of action. His only real concern was for my social life. He asked me how I would deal with the possibility of losing the friends I had made in my own age group.

My immediate reply was, "What friends?" I continued, "The only person I know well lives near me, and even we don't hang around together all that often. Most of the kids I know in this school are a grade ahead of me anyway. I mean, I'm already in some grade nine classes, so I know a lot of people in that grade; and they're the ones who are friendly to me. And I don't have a social life to speak of, so skipping a grade isn't going to make a difference that way. I really have nothing to lose. And besides, I have wanted to skip a grade since I was six years old. I should have been allowed to skip grade one, so it's about time."

By the end of the eighth grade school year, Meg, Lise and I had pretty much gone our separate ways. That I had no friends was absolutely true, and my acquaintances were, in fact, older than I. By skipping the ninth grade, I would actually be ahead socially. At least I hoped so.

My parents and the school principal gave me the go ahead. Then my whole world changed dramatically.

My dad was an industrial contractor who ran his own business for most of the '70s. Because of the uncertain political climate in Quebec at that time, the business closed. My family talked things over, and we decided to move to Denmark. Without going into too much detail, we moved to Denmark at the end of June 1978 and lived there until the end of September of that same year. Unfortunately, we could not adjust to the new lifestyle. It was just too different.

In Denmark my sisters and I were really messed up regarding our schooling. After my first week in class I refused to go to school at all. I was acutely aware that there was no way I could graduate high school in Denmark if I had to learn both grade ten work and fluent Danish in one year. The American assigned to teach Wanda and me Danish looked exactly like a substitute teacher I had had at The Asylum. I remember telling my family that I felt sure I knew this teacher from Montreal. I knew I did not want to attend his class—or any class at the Danish high school. The kids at school were not friendly towards me at all, and I was far too sad to put in any kind of effort towards making new friends, anyway. Depressed about both my educational situation and my social prospects, I opted to wallow in my misery. Instead of going to school, I stayed at home in my bed day in and day out. All I wanted was to return to my real home. I wanted to go back to Montreal.

My braces were removed while my family was in Denmark, so I would be going home with a big, beautiful smile on my face. And we did return home to Montreal . . . where I began to smoke.

The first week of October I started grade ten at my old high school. Since I was one month behind in my studies, I had to work extra hard to catch up; but I did not mind the work. Not at all. The only real disappointment I had relating to school was that I was relegated to playing the clarinet in band class for the second year in a row. Had I been present at the start of the school year in September, I would have chosen the saxophone. Oh well. It was still great to be back.

My favorite pastime when I was 14 years old was playing pinball. My family now lived in a large two-story apartment located across the street from the arcade. Going to the arcade every day after school was first a hobby, then an addiction. I would play pinball for hours at a time, leaving the arcade only at closing time. And it was at the arcade where I made some real friends—and where I had my first real obsession with a member of the opposite sex, Simon. My prior silent crushes were crushes. Meeting Simon, I graduated from silent crushes to silent obsessions. But he liked me as a friend only, the story of my life.

I do not know what happened or why, but during tenth grade I started cutting classes regularly. Although I kept up with homework and tests, I seldom attended class. For whatever reasons, I was happiest when rebelling against the system. Now that I had been promoted a grade level—the very thing I had wanted since I was 6 years old—I was no longer interested in school at all. My grades dropped a little, but I did not fare too badly considering I was in class approximately two thirds of the required time.

My rebelliousness did not extend to doing drugs. Forever concerned with keeping my "little gray cells" intact, as Agatha Christie's "Hercule Poirot" might say, I refused drugs completely. That is, I would not even take drugstore pharmaceuticals. I was not, however, averse to having a glass of wine or a couple of beers. And (like I need to say this) I smoked.

Do you remember Charlie? Charlie from my first elementary school? Charlie who loved Neil Young?

I did not . . . at the time.

In my tenth grade Canadian history classroom I sat next to a boy named Lenny. Lenny and I got along famously. Neither one of us paid any attention to the teacher, for one thing. This teacher had lost my respect and attention on the first day of class when he informed the class that the highest grade he would award anyone was an 85 percent. In other words, students who made no mistakes would receive a mark of 85 percent. Entirely disenchanted with this teacher's tactics, I did as little as was required to pass, and nothing more.

I regularly helped Lenny cheat on class assignments and tests. Throughout my life classmates asked me for help with their schoolwork, but I caught on early that these requests came from people who wanted to use me. And I do not appreciate being used. So invariably when asked for help, I answered, "No, sorry." It was different with Lenny. He was more of a rebel than I, and I liked him for that very reason. No one I knew at school could understand my bond with Lenny. *I* did not understand my bond with Lenny. Not really.

I made the link between Charlie and Lenny in 1990 when I recalled that they had the same surname. By grade ten, Charlie was going by the name Lenny. This first-name change explained why the history professor kept asking if "Charlie," rather than "Lenny," were present during roll call. I remember Lenny's usual response to roll call: "My name is Lenny now, man. I don't answer to 'Charlie' anymore."

I have no idea whether Lenny remembered me from way back when. If he did, he was playing The Game. But in all fairness, at the time I did not recognize him either.

Throughout grade ten I suffered from depression, which I attributed to regular teenage angst. I know that I was sad about not having a boyfriend (I never did have a boyfriend during my high school years), but the hopelessness I felt at that time went much deeper than whether or not I could get a date. It was more of a "What's the point?" type of despair. At age 14, I was thinking about life and the bigger picture. I had always pondered the meaning of it all, but never so profoundly as I did at this age. Wanting to know and understand why God had made me was foremost in my mind, especially considering that I felt so much sadness so much of the time.

> *All in time, it will be*
> *What it appears to seem to me*
> *All along, it's been said*
> *Live your life, you'll end up dead.*

> *Excerpt from poem "Pointless" © 1994, J. M. Knudsen*

I wrote these lines while deeply manic. Although the poem is too morose for my liking, it does embody my teenage philosophy on life. Everyone used to ask me why I was so negative when I was 14. My typical response: "Why not?"

I feel sure that much of my sadness at this age existed because faces from the baseball game—from the murder—were constantly surrounding me at school and at play. I did not know "who" these faces were at the time, but I know now that I must have made the connection between their faces and Sherry's murder in my subconscious. That The Game was in full swing during my tenth grade school year, 1978-79, is obvious to me now. And The Game's existence at my school explains why I felt such an urgent need to cut classes all of the time. In fact, I cut classes more and more as the school year dragged on. My teachers were well aware that I was skipping school, but they never reported me to the principal. I actually worked out special arrangements with four of my seven teachers wherein they would not report my absenteeism as long as I completed the assignments and tests and performed well. These teachers gave me a carte blanche, so to speak, and I therefore respected them and did as they asked.

Did I have any manic symptoms at age 14? Yes . . . I was obsessed with pinball. Addiction and obsession are one and the same, to me, and I was absolutely addicted to pinball. Also, when I did do schoolwork, I would complete three months' worth of assignments in one weekend. Having my freedom was and is paramount. To this day I hate obligations, even if the obligations are self-imposed. I am always setting deadlines for the projects I undertake. *I do not want to do things, so much as I want things done.*

And with that one sentence, I think I just described the very heart of mania. While I am being analytical, I will delve into mania further. Most manic people perpetually have several projects in mind, all of which require completion as soon as possible. Actually, mania is more of an "as soon as impossible" state of mind. Manics cannot possibly live up to their own expectations, so ultimately they crash and burn. And do they ever crash.

Manic depression is a lot like cross-country skiing. For those unfamiliar with the sport, cross-country skiing involves arduous climbing periods combined with occasional downhill moments until you reach the top of the mountain. Once at the top, you know the way becomes all downhill, all easy and all fun. The depression is akin to the climbing part of the skiing wherein you work your butt off for two seconds of fun. You climb and climb, and you finally reach the top of a puny, little hill; and then you get to slide down that hill for two whole seconds. Whoopee. The payoff seems nowhere in sight, and you find yourself wondering why you ever wanted to climb the damned mountain to begin with. But you do reach the top, eventually—and then you are manic. You know the way is all good from there: fast, furious and fun. And you know you will ski down that mountain in about one quarter of the time that it took you to climb it. The downhill skiing is a real rush. It is exhilarating! You never want this part of the skiing to end. But it does come to an end. You do reach the bottom of the mountain, again, putting you right back where you started; only now you have already climbed that mountain. To climb this mountain again would not give you the same thrill and sense of accomplishment. The mountain conquered, your purpose is gone and you crash hard. The mania has ended and left you without a direction, without a goal. And in your mind you hear, "It's finished. It's ended. Why did I bother?" And the crash at the bottom of the mountain is worse than the depression experienced while climbing it. So that is manic depression. Sort of.

Chapter 10

In June grade ten came to an end. Around this same time my dad was offered and accepted a job in Houston, Texas. I was totally excited at the prospects of a new city and new friends. My Montreal friends threw me a going-away party whereat the boy with whom I was enamored, Simon, kissed me goodbye. Oddly enough, the kiss did not live up to my expectations, and it therefore helped me to move on and to get over him.

When my family arrived in Houston in August 1979, the temperature was 100°F . . . in the shade. Right away I thought, "What have we done?" The heat made it difficult for me to breathe and, hypochondriac that I am, I thought I might drop dead on the spot. All of a sudden I was longing for the cooler climate of Canada, the "leather jacket weather," as I call it.

Upon arriving at our ranch-style home located in a nice suburb of Houston, I felt that things might be all right after all. The house, and pretty much every building in Texas, had built-in air conditioning. Outside it was very green and lush, which truly surprised me as I had expected the tumbling tumbleweeds one sees in westerns. Instead, I found myself in a tropical-like place complete with high humidity, lizards, locusts and *giant* cockroaches. Eek!

Our neighbors were friendly. Immediately, they came over to

our house and introduced themselves to us. This friendliness boded well for us in the social department, or so I hoped.

When Wanda and I went to enroll in the high school near our home, I convinced the counselor to place me in grade twelve. I explained to him that had I remained in Quebec, I would have been graduating that year, because Montreal's high schools only went to grade eleven. After going over the list of subjects that I had already studied in Montreal, the counselor agreed that I belonged in grade twelve. To be bypassing another year of high school pleased me no end. Hah! Double hah!

Childish? Well, I reserve the right to gloat when I beat the system. It is a rarity, after all.

I enjoyed grade twelve immensely. I had a near-perfect attendance record that year. Striving for 100%s in every class, I succeeded for the most part. I particularly enjoyed my world history class because the teacher was brilliant, thus inspiring me to learn and to work harder. Driver's education class was another plus in the Texas school system. I received my driver's license the day I turned 16.

As a senior in high school I had privileges: one free period a day, permission to leave the school grounds at lunch hour and exemption from final exams based on a combination of grades and absenteeism (an "A" in a given subject entitled you to four absences, a "B" entitled you to three misses, and so on). I relished all these freedoms. I chose first period as my free period because, like any other teenager, I wanted to sleep in. And I showed up for class every day because I had the incentive to do so.

On the downside—why is there always a downside?—smoking and the possession of tobacco were strictly prohibited on school grounds. I therefore began to chain-smoke at home. Somehow the number of cigarettes I smoked in a day increased that year, probably because I was smoking ultra-lights. Whatever.

Being a 15-year-old in grade twelve, I did not make many friends at school. Although I did not advertise my age to my fellow students, I am fairly certain they knew that I was younger. No matter. The seniors in school were 18 years old on average and had already established their social groups. Even if I had been older, I do not believe I would have been included in their circles.

Friendless and 15, I developed the philosophy that it was safer not to know people, that it was safer not to love people too much. Were I to keep to myself and just be alone all the time, no one could hurt me. When I say "alone," I really mean alone, but for my family.

I got the surprise of my life on my first day in twelfth grade when I bumped into a girl whom I recognized from Montreal. Liv had attended that same first Protestant elementary school where I had studied. She immediately acknowledged me and was friendly—for about five minutes. Perhaps she told everyone my age. I do not know. Maybe Liv was a player, maybe, but I doubt that The Game had reached Houston at this time.

By spring 1980 I finally found a real friend. Andrea was in grade ten and we hit it off right away. We talked on the phone for hours at a time. We socialized by going to movies, by shopping and by eating out. Andrea was probably the best female friend I ever had. I trusted her enough to help her with her schoolwork without experiencing the nasty feeling that I was being used. All in all, I was pretty happy in Houston, away from the players and the bad memories, away from the stress of The Game. I actually wore clothing in an assortment of colors that were not in the black family.

Yeah, I know you hear the "but." Life is just one great big "but" after another.

I received some terrible news in spring of 1980. My guidance counselor informed me that I was short 2 gym credits—yes, I said, "*gym credits*"—and that I would not be allowed to graduate in May with my class. I could not believe it! GYM? What the . . . (expletives deleted—there are just too many of them that apply here) . . . did gym have to do with my academic abilities? Nothing! This blow hit me hard. Not only did I conclude that hard work does not pay off, but also I realized that planning for the future is futile. Utterly, completely, absolutely futile!

Generally, I am a patient person. I take things in stride and I let the future take care of itself. But in this one instance I decided to fight. I was not going to let something as ridiculous as a couple of gym credits ruin my academic future. I therefore asked my high school principal to draft a letter explaining that I had, in fact, completed the grade twelve *academic* requirements (but for the 2 gym credits) and that I would be a good candidate for any university. A copy of his letter accompanied the three university applications I sent out. To my overwhelming joy and relief, I was accepted at one: Houston Baptist University.

I did not go to my high school prom. I could not go to commencement. But I did win a medal for earning the highest grade in my biology class, and accordingly I received an invitation to the awards ceremony. My mom insisted on getting me a special dress for the ceremony, and now I am happy that she did. Going to that ceremony was my goodbye to high school; it was my commencement. I knew my parents were proud of me, and I was kind of proud of myself. And happy. Knowing I would be starting university in a few months more than made up for any high school-related disappointments I may have endured.

High school ended in May 1980. In June, Wanda and I flew to Montreal to visit our grandparents for ten days. We had a great time in our hometown, except that we did not manage to meet with any of our former friends. I know that I was somewhat disappointed by this estrangement. However, Montreal is a beautiful city with much to see and do, and Wanda and I had a blast! Before we left Montreal, my grandmother gave me enough money to buy myself an old car in which I could commute to and from university. Upon returning to Texas, I bought a big, old, silver-gray car that I loved as though it were a Mercedes Benz.

Back in Houston, I could not wait to start university. Attending my first class in HBU at the end of August, I felt that I had finally arrived. I was 15 years old, I was a university freshman, and I had my own wheels. I was free, free, free at last! Attending university was my decision and not a requirement. That higher education was my choice made all the difference to my psyche. I *wanted* to go to class each day. I *wanted* to perform well. (And a part of me wanted to show "them" that I was worthy.)

Houston Baptist University is a private university that offers small, intimate class sizes; superior, caring instructors; and a safe, friendly environment. It was the ideal place for a 15-year-old who wanted to take on the world.

What . . . am I Mary Tyler Moore now?

In my entire life, I was never as happy in school as I was in HBU. It was a school wherein students could ask questions of their professors. Indeed, the professors encouraged their students to question, to argue, to think. The class sizes were small enough that the instructors knew their students by name. I know I felt that my teachers at HBU cared not only about my academic performance but also about me, Janet. If I should one day find myself in a position to continue my university studies, I will go back to HBU.

I chose business administration as my field with accounting as my major. Law school was my ultimate goal. I made the dean's list that first term and all subsequent terms. By exam, I was awarded 12 French credits. Having been educated in Quebec for the most part, I had no difficulties passing the advanced-placement French test. I made friends with the smoking crowd, as we naturally gravitated towards each other. Even as far back as 1980, many Texans frowned upon smoking and rightfully so.

Who said that? It couldn't have been me, puff, puff, puff. OK, the part of me that's logical knows smoking is a bad thing. But cigarettes are essential props in order to achieve that "affected artist" look.

HBU operated using a quarter system wherein 36 credits per school year were considered a full-time study program. Having earned 12 French credits off the bat, I decided to take off the second term and work for tuition money. The tuition was high enough, and I did not feel that my parents should be solely responsible for the cost of my education. Besides, I was now 16 and had never worked a day in my life. I wanted to see what work was like. And I wanted stuff; specifically, I wanted my very own stereo system.

In general, I am not a person who wants much of anything. I do not collect things because I do not care for clutter. A running automobile, guitars, food, shelter and clothing are all that I require. Anything beyond these items is clutter, stuff. At 16, I guess I was still in my greedy phase wherein I equated success with money. (Happily,

I outgrew that type of thinking.) I found a full-time job in a department store and worked there from November 1980 to March 1981. Oh, and I did buy myself a stereo.

Yet another dramatic blow . . .

At the end of March my dad decided to leave his job in Houston and move our family back to Montreal. When I tried to transfer to a university in Montreal, I was told that in addition to my 21 credits from HBU, I would require 9 more university credits and calculus to do so. Thirty credits were the standard minimum requirement to transfer schooling from one university to another in Canada. I was screwed. Montreal's school system did it to me again. And once more, I found myself pondering the futility of planning anything in life. My cynicism returned stronger than ever.

When I think about Texas, I have nothing but good, happy thoughts. Texans encourage success and reward hard work. When a roadblock appears, they determine a workable detour. Canada has almost always let me down in terms of education and employment. I am happy to be a Canadian, but I wish this country would do more for its students. In Canada it is difficult to transfer schooling from one province to another. It is somewhat akin to moving a mountain to transfer schooling from another country to Canada. Why? Why are entrance rules more important than are students? Why is compromise nonexistent?

I am happy—lucky—that my illness surfaced now that I am in Canada. We do have a wonderful health care system, and our doctors and nurses are dedicated, intelligent individuals. But I really wish someone, somewhere, would challenge our schooling methods and come up with a more accessible system.

So ends my rant.

Since I was unable to transfer to a university in Montreal, I looked for and was lucky to find employment with a major magazine company in June 1981. I was hired to work in the complaints department (yes, I see the irony there), but I soon found my own niche doing departmental reports and statistics. A friend of mine from tenth grade, Cindy, applied for a job with the company and was hired partially on my recommendation. I was quite pleased about that. The nicest group of people with whom I have ever had the pleasure to work was the group at this magazine company.

In July my friend Andrea flew from Houston to Montreal to visit me for a couple of weeks. She loved Montreal. She said it was the "nicest, most fun place" she had ever been. Andrea and I did all the tourist things; in fact, we visited buildings, parks and churches that *I* had not seen before. It was a fun time.

The drudgery of office work got to me after about eight months on the job. I could not foresee a happy future being an office clerk forever. When my boss told me that I was in line for a promotion, my response was not as it should have been. Instead of this news giving me joy, I felt like a caged animal. I had to escape this job, and fast!

And when I search I find that
The game's the same . . .

Excerpt from song "Around the Block" © 1990, J. M. Knudsen

In addition to my high school friend, I had another pal at work named Angie. Angie's boyfriend, whom she discussed with me on occasion, was named Nick. One day out of the blue, Nick came to our office cafeteria to have lunch with Angie. I did not recognize Nick at the time. He had dyed his hair platinum blonde and he now sported a crew cut. Nick, Lenny and Charlie were one and the same. For purposes of this book, I will say that his last name was "Jones." Mr. Jones. I like that. It works for me.

I realize I wanted out of my job pretty much around the time Nick first came to lunch. I fell for Nick instantly, but there was no way I would ever go after another girl's boyfriend as I always thought it classless to interfere with another person's relationships. Still do. Anyway, I can now see that The Game was ongoing and that Nick was a player. When Angie introduced me to Nick, he acted as though we had never met before. I certainly did not recognize or remember him. It had been over three years since my high school days with Lenny, and in my traumatized state I did not recognize any person involved with Sherry's murder if more than a year had elapsed between meetings.

Seeing Nick meant The Game was real and ongoing. Depression set in anew. I did not relate this sadness to Nick, however, because I was not yet consciously aware of The Game.

What did Nick want? What was The Game? He questioned me endlessly about music. He wanted to know which bands I favored, what concerts I had attended and whether I played any instruments myself.

I told Nick that I loved The Rolling Stones and Rod Stewart and that I played guitar. I had just recently bought a blue electric guitar and an amplifier with the money I had saved from working. Nick thought that was "cool." I also told him that I had been fortunate to see Rod Stewart in concert in February 1982 and then added that Tom Petty was my current favorite. Nick pounced on that statement. He said, "Why don't we go to see Tom Petty when he plays here? He's coming in a couple of weeks, man."

I assumed "we" meant Angie, Nick and me, and I told Nick that I would be interested in going. My conversation with Nick seemed to upset Angie. I do not know whether she was in on The Game, but I do know I liked her. I thought perhaps Nick was using her to get to me. Nick came to lunch at work a few more times, and the three of us did go to see Tom Petty as planned.

When I became sick in 1990 and began to unravel Sherry's murder and The Game, I wanted to believe the best about Mr. Jones. I had loved him from a very young age and wanted so much for him to be on my side. But I now concede that seeing Nick, Lenny, Charlie Jones for the third time without his admitting to having known me in the past meant he was a player. Perhaps even the puppet master.

Chapter 11

In June 1982 I decided to return to Houston Baptist University to obtain the 9 credits that I required to gain entrance into a Montreal university. After having discussed my academic situation at great length with the admissions officer in Montreal, I learned that with 9 more credits I could transfer to the arts program. Once I had completed the calculus requirement at night school, I could then transfer to the business administration program. I was willing to bend. I was willing to do whatever it took to get back into school and finish my degree.

I called my friend Andrea in Texas and asked her if I could stay at her house for the first five-week summer term of 1982. Not only did her family take me into their home, but they also lent me the use of a vehicle with which to commute to and from school.

I was somewhat sad to leave my job at the magazine company. However, as things never go as planned, my dad received a lucrative job offer in Fort McMurray, Alberta, in January 1982; and he immediately left Montreal to go and work in that small northern town. In July, while I was studying in Houston, my mom and my sisters joined my dad in Fort McMurray. Given that I was not yet ready to make it on my own, I would have left my job anyway. Regardless, I had no intention of letting this latest move stop me from going to university in Montreal. My grandmother would take me in to live with her as required, and I would fly back and forth to Fort McMurray whenever possible.

Around the second week of June I flew to Houston. This time the heat did not seem unbearable. This time I really wanted to be there. I signed up for three, 3-credit classes to be completed in an intensive, five-week session. Once again the Texas school system worked with me, not against me. Although the maximum class load for a summer term was 6 credits, the school made an exception for me and allowed me to go for the 9 credits that I required. The summer session's intensive study program was completely suited to my nature, my "get it done yesterday" attitude. I worked hard that term and got straight As for my effort. I also had a wonderful time hanging out with Andrea. In the end, I did not want to leave, but I could not afford to stay.

I wrote my final exams and left Houston around the middle of July. The apprehension I felt when leaving Houston was palpable. I had no idea what to expect from Fort McMurray. The only thing I knew about this city was that it was small. Very small. I thought—hoped—it would be a good, friendly place in which to live. Throughout my life I had heard that small towns are friendlier than the large cosmopolitan cities to which I was accustomed. Oh well.

You just know this ain't going to be good.

I got off the plane in Fort McMurray, and my parents drove me to our new home. I remember saying and thinking one thought only: "I'm in 'Lumberland'."

Depression entered into my life as never before. Somehow, I could not foresee making friends in this town. Not into camping, fishing or any other outdoor activities, I felt certain that I would not fit in here. That the Fort McMurray locals lived for these types of pastimes was readily apparent.

Prior to my leaving Houston, Andrea and I made plans for her to come and visit me in my new home. So at least I could look forward to her visit, a visit I should have canceled considering my feelings towards this small town. Andrea arrived in Fort McMurray within a few weeks of my arrival. Our friendship fell apart during her visit. I was angry at the world, and I took it out on everyone in sight.

Too depressed to entertain anyone, I just wanted to wallow in my own self-pity. I think I almost hated Andrea because I was envious of her. She would be going back to Houston in a few weeks, whereas I would be stuck in Fort McMurray for God knows how long. At the earliest, I would have to wait until January '83 to transfer to the university in Montreal.

Back in Texas, Andrea wrote me a scathing letter, and I deserved every anger-filled word of it. I never answered that letter. I remember thinking, "Why bother. You won't see her again anyway." To this day, the situation with Andrea weighs upon my conscience. I am sorry for treating her badly. Truly sorry.

Depression encompasses more than just sadness. It often manifests itself in the guise of anger. When in the throes of depression, I often used to lash out at the people I loved most. I wanted to hurt them so that they could feel what I was feeling. It was as though I blamed them for my unhappiness. My logic was skewed: I thought if people were happy, they must be doing something wrong, because I was miserable and I was not hurting anyone. As I grew older, I realized that the anger and depression were connected. Once I established this link, when in my depressed states, I no longer attacked those I loved. Instead I began to tell myself, "I'm angry because I'm sad and it's nobody's fault. Let it go."

I mailed off my transfer application to the university in Montreal in August '82, fully expecting to be accepted for admission to the January 1983 term.

Woe and alas! I plannethed in vain once again. Hath they no mercy for this downtrodden lass? Do they not knoweth the damage they wreaketh?

The futility of planning hit hard this time. My reply from the Montreal university stated that I would require 12 additional credits to transfer to their renowned halls. According to their letter the 12 French credits that I had been awarded by exam in Houston were nontransferable. I telephoned the admissions office in Montreal to argue my case. I explained to the admissions official that I had *already* discussed my situation with an officer at their school and that, at considerable expense to me, I had done exactly what I was told to do in order to transfer. (Between the flight and the tuition my term in Houston was costly.) The official responded that the university was sorry for the oversight but that they would be happy to admit me once I obtained those missing 12 credits. I wanted to say "Fuck it!" but instead I held my tongue and softly said, "Goodbye."

Now what? Everything I had worked for was history. I really did not know how to proceed with my life now that my plans had been utterly destroyed. Luckily, my dad had a solution. He suggested that I could work for a little while and think about school again once I was calmer. In addition, he reminded me that there were other universities and that I did not have to go to the one in Montreal. Although I had never entertained the idea of studying elsewhere, I had to agree with my dad. I could apply to universities in Alberta and British Columbia, and in the interim I could work and save for my tuition.

In October 1982 I was hired as an apprentice insulator at one of Fort McMurray's oil sands plants. Being a union apprentice, I was paid extremely well. I was paid so well that I almost decided to forget about university altogether, but deep down I knew I could not foresee myself insulating in the long run.

That same month I took out an ad in the local newspaper that stated, "Rhythm guitar player seeks band." A lead guitar player named Rob telephoned me immediately. He said that he knew a drummer and a bass player and that he could arrange for us to meet. I was thrilled! Maybe life in Fort McMurray would be better than I had originally anticipated. The three musicians showed up at my house the next evening, and we discussed our musical preferences and goals. We agreed to be a heavy metal band and began practicing in my basement that same week. Even though I was not a metal aficionado, I wanted to be in a band badly; so I compromised. I wrote a metal song called *Trusting Child* that was eventually published in the HBU writers magazine. I also wrote a folk-rock song called *The Key*, which remains a favorite of mine to this day.

The Key

I don't know where I've been, nor what is to become of me
Time will tell, it's all to see
What the future holds for me

I don't know who you are, nor how you made it here so far
What's your secret to success
Who're you trying to impress

What you make in life is yours, it's your choice to close the
doors
Happiness can be achieved
But it's up to you to find the key

But there are changes coming through, and I smile when I
see you
Lights are shining in the sky—shining bright, we're on a new
high

Long away down on the road, there's a place I long to be
I keep searching endlessly
Fulfillment is that which I seek

Life surprises us all
One can never really tell
What tomorrow holds in store
Certainly we know no more
Than we ever knew before.

Song "The Key" © 1982, J. M. Knudsen

The meaning of this song completely eluded me at the time.
No sooner did I meet my drummer, Tristan, than I developed
a crush on him. He was 6'2" with eyes of blue, with long curly brown
locks and with a winning smile. As was my wont, I kept my feelings

to myself. I reasoned that if Tristan liked me, he would let me know; otherwise, we would be friends. At 18, I thought this was the adult way to deal with the situation. Anyway, my feelings for Tristan amounted to a crush, not an obsession. In fact, at this time I also had my eye on a young man from work named Sean.

A girlfriend of mine from work arranged for Sean and me to meet one night at a bar. She was supposed to meet us there, but she never showed up. Sean and I had a nice time, regardless. I was aware that he was a "stoner"—that he often smoked marijuana—but he was nice and fun, and he could make me laugh. Suffice to say, I was willing to overlook his bad habits. After our initial date, Sean and I got together a few more times at his house. Basically, we listened to music while he got stoned. There was no physical side to this relationship because he was *always* stoned. His room was adorned with typical occult paraphernalia: skulls, candles, incense and . . . a rather large satanic bible. I questioned him about this book. He said that he had bought it to "freak people out" and that he did "not take it seriously."

During the Christmas season I asked Sean to accompany me to a house party being hosted by friends of my parents. I had one beer when I arrived. My second drink was a gin and tonic that Sean made for me. I had had no more than two sips of this drink when the room began to spin and I became violently ill. Immediately I told my mom that I was feeling sick. Neither my mom nor I could understand why. Two drinks were not unusual for me, and I was in the habit of spacing out my drinks at one per hour.

Did Sean put something in my drink? If he did, could that drug be the root of my paranoid delusions? I have heard in the news lately that the drug "ecstasy" can induce psychotic traits in some cases. Was I slipped a similar drug? I know I suffered no delusions or hallucinations prior to this party. (I did not remember Sherry or anything to do with her murder, so none of that paranoia was playing into my life at this time—I was sane.)

In the following weeks and months, I started to phase out now and then. I would find myself staring at a light or at some object that had caught my eye, with no thoughts in my head, just spaced out.

And then I would come to and wonder what had happened. I mean, I knew that I had been staring at some object, but I could not for the life of me figure out why. And when I did come to, it was like I had just awakened from a deep sleep, like I had been hypnotized. I could hear my family talking to me while I was in these trances, but their voices seemed distant. I would respond to them sometimes as much as ten minutes after they had last spoken to me. My brain was working in slow motion. I did not realize that a time lapse had existed between their statements and my responses. My behavior was so strange that my mom eventually asked me if I were on drugs. I responded that I had never taken drugs and never would. My mom believed me, but still she was perturbed by my spaced-out behavior. After a few months I was back to normal, and my temporary trances were soon forgotten.

The boys in the band and I frequented the local nightclubs on weekends. We were particularly interested in seeing live bands, checking out the competition.

It was the strangest thing. In January 1983 I hailed a cab to take me home from a nightclub. The cab driver looked at me and said, "You are a musician. You will be world famous as a solo guitar player. Please remember my words."

The cab driver had no way of knowing that I was a musician; I had not played publicly. So I responded, "As a solo? That's not possible. I have to have a band with me. I don't have the nerve to play alone. At least not in public."

"Solo!" And he spoke the word with such finality that I did not argue the point any further. I really thought that he was way off in his prediction, but I did resolve to work on my solo playing after our meeting.

My band practiced three or four times a week to no avail, although in February Rob and I did play a duet on the local television station as part of a charity drive. Can you imagine? My very first public performance in which I sang and played the guitar was televised. I was a nervous wreck!

You know what's funny? The first song Rob and I played that night was "Heart of Gold" by Neil Young. I hope that makes up for anything negative I may have thought when I was a kid.

I also sang my song *The Key* and it was well received. I had no confidence in my songwriting abilities at this time, so I was ecstatic upon discovering that people liked my song, my original. Even with this audience acceptance, I did not write another song until 1990. I think the breakup of my band rendered me somewhat disenchanted with music for a while. Oh well. The band was destined to go nowhere right from the start. We could not agree on who should be the singer, and Tristan was a drummer without rhythm. Neither I nor the other members of the band had the heart to replace our drummer. Ultimately, all of us as a group agreed to disband. There was no one to blame and no hard feelings. After the breakup, Tristan and I got together one night and drank wine and . . . he was my first love. That was what I wanted, and so I was happy.

During our time together the guys in my band threw many parties at the house they had rented for the purpose of practicing. Mr. Jones and his band were present at two of these parties. Still, I did not know who Mr. Jones was. We met "for the first time" for the fourth time. He asked me to look at some of his song lyrics because he wanted my opinion. "Too cliché" was my response.

In spring the guys in the band went their separate ways. I think Tristan moved to British Columbia, and the bass player moved back to Ontario. Rob joined another band and left town.

I was heartbroken. I was alone again.

Greta Garbo was born on September 18th just like me. I find it hard to believe she "wanted to be alone," but I do understand waiting for true love and the unwillingness to settle for anything less.

No friends and stuck in a piss-ant town. But I did have a brand new car! In my year at the plant I saved enough money to buy myself a new car and a twelve-string guitar. I could adjust to life in this town; I *would* adjust to life in this town. Being friendless once more, I decided the time was opportune for me to work on both my singing and my guitar playing.

When the boys in the band left town, Wanda and I signed up for karate lessons in the hopes of meeting new people. We did not. We did, however, succeed in earning our yellow belts.

I stayed at the plant until October 1983. After having worked there for a year, I was bored out of my skull. It was time for a change. (My whole life has been nothing but changes, but I guess that is what keeps it interesting.) I opted to go back to Houston Baptist University and get the 12 credits I required to transfer to the Montreal university. Yes, I said, "the Montreal university." I would give it one more try.

Having put together sufficient funds, I flew to Texas for the spring term of 1984. This time I stayed in the school dormitory, and this time I was really on my own. There were no friends upon whom I could call—I dared not phone Andrea. Fortunately, I was housed in a room with a girl who smoked, and we got along well. I also befriended a medical student named Glenn whom I met in my English class. He and I had a lot in common and are friends to this day. I related well to Glenn because he, too, had skipped a grade in high school. (And I thank him for finding me a television set when I was rooming on my own during the summer sessions.)

It was my English professor at HBU who inspired me to write this book. She praised my writing; indeed, she tried to persuade me to change my major to English. To receive encouragement from such a brilliant lady was heartwarming. Her words of encouragement never left me.

I thought I saw Mr. Jones at a party in Houston one night that spring. I wrote in my diary, "I just met the man of my dreams . . ." But I could be wrong.

I earned straight As for the spring term and was awarded a small scholarship for my efforts. As it was the only scholarship available to foreign students, I was quite pleased to have earned it. Given the scholarship, I asked my parents if I could remain in Houston for the two summer terms as well. They consented immediately. All in all, I earned 24 credits during this stay in Houston—more than enough credits to transfer to the Montreal university or to any Canadian university, for that matter.

I was sad to leave Texas in mid-August. However, I missed my family terribly.

Even the best laid plans blah blah blah . . .

When I returned to Fort McMurray, I immediately went to visit the local branch office of an Alberta correspondence university and left the office with three classes in hand. Knowing that I could not go to the Montreal university until January '85, I decided to take correspondence classes in the interim. I did not want to take yet another break from my studies.

I quickly discovered that I had no more than two weeks to submit an application to the university in Montreal. Time was of the essence, so I flew to Montreal the first week of September to expedite my application and to ensure my acceptance for the January '85 semester. Three days later, I returned to Fort McMurray.

Within a week I received the reply to my application. This refusal notice informed me that I had "insufficient transfer credits" and that I "lacked calculus," which was now a requirement to all programs at the school. Apparently some of the classes I had studied in Houston were now nontransferable.

I cried—and I conceded defeat, but not before I wrote a scathing letter to the university describing both my ordeal and my opinion of their admissions policies. I would never again attempt to go to this school. They had succeeded in breaking my spirit, for a while.

My next step was to apply to a university in Edmonton, Alberta. If I had to leave Fort McMurray to go to university, then I wanted to be as close to my family as possible. I was refused entrance to the Edmonton university for reasons much the same as those touted by the Montreal university. I believe I lacked "nine credits . . ."

When one door closes, another opens . . .

It was time to change tactics. Having run myself ragged in my attempts to transfer to a Canadian university, I decided to take my complaints to a higher power. I wrote a lengthy letter to my local Member of Parliament explaining the myriad of difficulties I had experienced in trying to transfer to a university in my native land. Not only did the Member of Parliament read my letter in session in the nation's capital, Ottawa, but also he procured my acceptance to a university in Calgary, Alberta.

Whereas I gripe about the problems I have encountered with Canada's educational system, I have nothing but praise for my country's political representation. On the three occasions where I turned to a politician for assistance, I received immediate, positive replies.

My acceptance to the Calgary university was a hollow victory. At best, I would have to work for a year to accumulate the means to study out of town. But I did feel happy knowing that a door had opened at long last. I decided my next best move was to sign up for more correspondence courses and hold off on going to Calgary until my finances improved. Oh, and I decided to take guitar lessons.

Chapter 12

In February 1985 I noticed an advertisement for a new music store located in my neighborhood in Fort McMurray. Given that the only other music store in town was grossly overpriced and somewhat impersonal, I headed over to this new store immediately. Although the store was small, with limited stock, the owner and assistant manager were so amiable that I resolved to frequent this new establishment for my future musical needs. And I decided I needed to take guitar lessons. My playing had reached a plateau that left me feeling unsatisfied and wanting. I knew there was so much more to learn. I knew, too, that I had to master the guitar.

I signed up to take guitar lessons from Al, the owner, and went to my first lesson that same week. After hearing me play, Al said that he could not really teach me anything that I did not already know; and he then asked me if I would be interested in a job as his assistant manager. His current assistant was leaving town in a month.

I was floored. For so long I had felt inferior in my playing ability, and now I was being offered a job because of my talent. My background in business administration, specifically bookkeeping, also played into Al's offer. I took a week to think it over. It was my dream job in every respect except for the salary, which was minimal, but it was an opportunity that I could not refuse.

I accepted the position and commenced working in the store

in March 1985. Within a month I bought myself an acoustic steel-string guitar of the six-string variety. I was fed up with the twelve-string guitar I had bought years earlier because it did not have the bass sound that I wanted. I could hear my sound in my head. All I had to do was figure out how to get this sound to come out on the guitar.

In my year working with Al, I learned a lot about guitar playing. The store had a fantastic selection of guitar music books, and I made it my mission to go through all of them. There was a fair bit of downtime at this job, time that I spent playing my instrument. Indeed, I was manic in my desire to learn everything I could about the guitar. Rock, finger-picking, flamenco, jazz, bluegrass, classical—I had to know all of these forms. Everything. Ultimately, I was playing guitar eight hours a day, learning, absorbing, improving and slowly devising my own sound, my own style.

Music is my life, man.

That guitar became my obsession is an understatement. I let my correspondence courses slide until I withdrew from my university studies altogether. I could no longer summon any interest in business classes when I knew that it was the guitar that gave me joy. And I am selfish. I embrace and cherish my bliss whenever and wherever I find it. Sustained bliss is a part of the good mania, after all, and I do enjoy the good mania. Who would not?

Working at the music store, I found my niche. I still wanted to put a band together, but I felt that that would happen when the time was right.

Not long after I began working in the music store, Al hired Daryl as a full-time guitar teacher and a part-time salesman. Daryl would mind the store on my days off. Daryl and I got along right away, and I found myself infatuated with him in no time. Again, as with Tristan, I kept my feelings to myself. By this time I had refined hiding my true feelings into an art form. Daryl and I spent much of our free time together, even keeping each other company at work on our days off. We were the best of friends, and Fort McMurray became bearable once again.

Daryl introduced me to different music. David Bowie and Prince stand out in my memory. As I had never really listened to

either of these musicians, I was shamefully ignorant of their music
and of their brilliance. Once I heard their music, however, I was
completely enamored of them. I bought every Bowie and Prince album
I could find. Their words, their music, manna from Heaven. That I
deem them musical geniuses goes without saying; in fact, I think they
are as brilliant today as were Mozart and Beethoven in their time.

*Of course, The Rolling Stones fall into the genius category
as well, but I knew of their genius at a much younger age. I wasn't a
total heathen prior to meeting Daryl.*

Even though I was content with my job and my friendship
with Daryl, I remember falling into a deep depression in the fall of
1985 that continued well into 1986. I was always telling Al that I
wanted "gray skies to suit my mood." Strangely, more often than not,
I got my gray skies. I recall Al one day asking me to wish for blue
skies, as though I had the power to change their color. But I was
simply too sad to oblige him. I continued to wish for my gray! The
depression was very real, the worst so far.

Vanity, thy name is woman.

When depressed, I become utterly obsessed with my
appearance. The obsessive traits became apparent in 1985.

The first trait to manifest itself was the "wearing of the black."
I always wore black clothing. At first I mixed black with other colors;
but the black was ever present, even if only my shoes were this darkest
of colors.

Another obsession was my hair. I dyed, permed, cut and grew
my hair continually. In 1985 the color of choice was red, specifically
fake red. I told my stylist I wanted a red that did not occur in nature.
I wanted people to know that my hair was dyed. I wanted to look
fake.

Weight was my final depression-related obsession. I slimmed
down to 115 lbs in '85, and I constantly felt a need to lose "just five
more pounds." Al jokingly began to call me "Ann," as in "anorexia."
Fortunately, I did not succumb to either anorexia or bulimia thanks to
my never-sated sweet tooth.

Why I was so depressed at this time, I do not know. Maybe it
was related to Daryl's viewing me as a friend only. That was part of it.

However, armed with the knowledge of Daryl's feelings towards me, I kept my eyes and heart open to the possibility of meeting someone new. I did not permit my feelings for Daryl to become an obsession. No, the depression I was feeling went deeper than the sorrow I felt because of unrequited love. It was the "hurt that had no name" depression. I cried all the time—at home. In public, I put on my happy face.

The happy face. The mask. I had trained myself to wear the mask at a very young age. My smile looked achingly sweet, but it was a smile nonetheless. I remember that I did not want people to see that I was sad. For some reason, I believed I had to keep my sorrow to myself—that if anyone knew, my world would collapse.

Al saw through the mask. At the time, he made a cryptic statement that I well recall: "Janet, I've known you for almost a year, but I don't feel like I know you at all."

I responded that I did not have a clue what he was talking about. I really did not.

Are we ready for more paranoia? More about The Game?

Daryl claimed to be from the Yukon Territory in northern Canada. He said that Fort McMurray and the Yukon were the only two places in which he had resided. But when I lost my grip on reality in 1990, I remembered having seen Daryl at my high school in Montreal. He was not in any of my classes; however, his locker was near mine, and we usually acknowledged each other with hellos. Knowing that Daryl was lying, that he had lived in Montreal, would certainly explain the mask I wore when around him. Paranoia. Maybe it is just paranoia. Do not know, cannot say.

In January 1986 Daryl proposed that I could join his rock band were I willing to play the synthesizer. He knew I could play the piano as I was teaching beginners piano at the store. Synthesizers were hot in the '80s. It seemed that every band had a synthesizer player, that it had become almost a requirement. So I bought a synthesizer. Boy, was I naïve.

The older I grew, the more aware I became that there was chauvinism in the music industry. I discovered that men, in general, had no qualms about women playing the piano; but when a woman played the guitar well, she was deemed a pariah, of sorts. The competitiveness and jealousy where the guitar was concerned were noticeable, tangible. Many men—and I emphasize *many,* not *all*—seemed to think that the guitar was their instrument and theirs alone. When did the guitar become the property of men only? After all, accomplished women played the lute way back when, and in the early 1900s there were many famous female blues and bluegrass guitar players. My contention is that the invention of the electric guitar signaled the beginning of the "guitar is for men only" attitude. The electric guitar allowed players to play louder than ever before, and volume is just so macho. Happily, attitudes have changed greatly since the '70s and '80s, and female guitar players now abound and are accepted.

The tirade has now ended. Please relax and enjoy the rest of the story.

Al said that he could not teach me anything about guitar playing. But he was wrong. He taught me the most important aspect of my playing, my style, today. He taught me *volume!* One day he was listening to me strum and sing, and he said, simply, "You need to play louder."

I agreed and complied. Al was a very wise man.

Daryl and I became closer and closer over time. He was the best friend I ever had, or so I thought. We spent our free time going to movies, restaurants and nightclubs together. Our outings felt like dates but without the romance. Daryl had one trait that I greatly appreciated: he danced. As I love dancing almost as much as I love playing the guitar and singing, he won my heart by his willingness to dance with me.

> *Into the night I go*
> *And dance and drink and lose control*
> *But it takes all these little things*
> *To get me on my feet again*
> *And it might just matter anyhow.*

Excerpt from song "Out of the Sky" © 1994, J. M. Knudsen

Dancing, like the guitar, cuts through all my sadness, all my despair, and makes me feel truly free. But guitar is first in my heart because it gives me something dancing cannot: a sense of accomplishment. Every time I learn a new song or perfect a difficult piece, I feel not only happy but also satisfied. Holding the guitar in my arms, I am at peace, at home. My guitars are my children; they are a part of me.

All good things must come to an end. Why, I ask you? Why? The oil sands boom in Fort McMurray went bust in the spring of 1986. All of a sudden there was no work to be had. Many of the city's residents, my family included, were now scurrying to sell their homes and move elsewhere. And during these trying times my beloved Grannie Ronnie came to Fort McMurray so that she could be with her family, with us, when she passed away. She had cancer and had been ill for quite some time. By April 1986 the fight had left her. With great dignity and grace, she accepted that she was dying.

I did not—could not—watch her waste away. I had never had to deal with the reality of death up close. I remember I gave her a powder-blue mohair sweater that I had knitted, and she wore it every day to fight off the chills that would not leave her body. That was all I could think to do. A sweater. She passed away on April 23, 1986. I did not cry at the time. I was too numb, too confused. She was my grandmother. She was not supposed to die. Not yet.

In life, Grannie Ronnie was a vivacious, happy, fun, religious lady. Although she was born in Newfoundland, a Maritime province, she was a Montrealer at heart. She loved the excitement of living in a big, bustling, cosmopolitan city. She was forever on the go. The downtown was her home more than any ocean could ever be. Grannie Ronnie would sing at the drop of a hat, and she loved to dance. Always advocating that money was meant to be spent, she did not save so much as a dime in her lifetime. What fun was there in having the money? Money was just paper, after all. No, she reasoned money was only as good as what you could buy with it, and she was right. She enjoyed life fully. Perhaps because she was not greedy and never worried about her tomorrows, she also lived her life freely. If I inherited the ability to do anything musical, I inherited it from her. I never picture her as she looked in her final days. I remember my Grannie Ronnie as a beautiful, happy, robust free spirit who understood life and God better than most people ever do or ever will. I loved her. I love her.

I quit my job at the music store at the end of April. My dad had decided that it was time to move, and he chose Edmonton as the city that would be our new home.

Chapter 13

Edmonton. I had wanted to move to Edmonton, Alberta, from day one in Fort McMurray; and now that my family was finally going to do so, I was not ready to go. I was tremendously saddened at the thought of leaving Daryl and being friendless once again. The arduous process of meeting new people was utterly unappealing to me. I had been through this process many times and knew from experience that real friends are few and far between.

We sold our house in Fort McMurray and moved to Edmonton, where I still reside, in June 1986. Within two weeks of our move Daryl came to visit me, and he and I were constantly in touch via the telephone. I realized that I could withstand living in Edmonton once I knew that Daryl and I would remain friends. I was definitely happier being in a big city. In fact, I was unaware of just how much I had missed city life until I settled into my new life in Edmonton.

Virtually upon arrival in the big city, I dyed my hair black for the first time. I had toyed with the idea of going black for a long time but had lacked the nerve to do so. Black hair makes a statement. Black hair tells people that you are your own person, that you are independent and not a slave to the opinions of others. To me, black hair is a sign of inner strength. Upon seeing myself with raven hair for the first time, I felt that strength, and I felt right. Ironically, no other hair color had cheered me up as much as did black. With my pale complexion and Cupid's bow lips, I looked like a porcelain doll. And for the first time in my life, I felt pretty. My mom, who is the most beautiful woman I know, had ultra-dark hair when she was young. I wanted to look like Mom.

Following the move and the newly adopted black hair, there was a noticeable change in Daryl's treatment of me. When we now visited each other, he would make occasional sexual advances towards me—advances that made me believe that our having a romantic, loving relationship was a future possibility. Advances that ultimately turned my crush into a mild obsession.

In July I decided to look for a job in the world-famous West Edmonton Mall. My family and I were living about five minutes away from this attraction, so it seemed like a good place to start my job search. A trendy clothing store hired me on the spot as a part-time sales clerk. I liked my job. More accurately, I liked my employee discount. But there was a downside.

There was a downside? No way!

Even though I worked with people in my own age group, I was not included in any of their many social outings. My coworkers— who sported the "Goth," or Gothic, look that includes black clothes, white-faced makeup, tattoos and piercings—were not interested in knowing me. I was not Goth. Despite my black hair, I was not Goth. Indeed, I was unacquainted with the alternative scene and its clothing and music altogether. My belief is that I was ostracized because I did not follow the group. I have never been a follower. I do what I do.

Around this time, I went to see Chrissie Hynde and the Pretenders in concert. I was overjoyed to see Chrissie because she was the first woman I knew of who played electric guitar and fronted her own band. She was living my dream, only I envisioned myself playing an acoustic six-string guitar.

My part-time job at the clothing store was short lived. When sales slowed down early in September, my hours were reduced to the point that I deemed quitting my only option. Once more I found myself scrambling for something new to do with my life. Since I had always loved travel, the idea of either becoming a stewardess or working for a cruise line appealed to me. Accordingly, I signed up for a six-month travel and tourism course at a downtown college and graduated at the top of my class. Despite sending out numerous applications, I was unsuccessful in finding a travel-related position. The only serious job offer I entertained required my relocating to Halifax, Nova Scotia. I was, however, unwilling to move so far away from my family and attempt to go it alone in a strange city.

So . . . I lied my way into a full-time job as a cocktail waitress for a pizza restaurant and lounge and started work in March 1987. A girl I had met in my travel course worked as a cocktail waitress and had told me the money was good in this field. She coached me sufficiently about waitressing that I could fake my way into a job and seem experienced.

I loved being a cocktail waitress. The tips were great and I was out every night. I found out that I loved the nightlife; I did not care if I saw daylight again. My job was my social life. I partied with my coworkers often, and regularly stayed at the lounge, which had a dance floor and a deejay, to dance following my shifts. My free nights were spent at the lounge, as well, because I had befriended many of my customers. Work was the place to be. My job was my joy . . . and my life.

Although I had experienced both manic and depressive tendencies in the past, it was not until I worked as a cocktail waitress that I became truly manic depressive. I believe the mania was an extension of the excitement and joy that stemmed from my new status of being part of a group, of having a social life and of discovering that men did find me attractive. I know the mania was very real. I could not sleep, and I was perpetually anxious to get back to work at the lounge where I was ecstatic whether working or playing. On the nights when I danced, I did so for two or more hours without a break. I was *never* tired, *never* too worn out to dance a little longer or to go to the next party. All-nighters were common.

I am diagnosed as being "atypical" bipolar. What that means is that I do not have the usual long-term bouts of mania or of depression. My manic phases typically last for a month or two, but they can be as short as a few days. The same applies to my depressive phases. Some might say I am lucky. To be on the endless roller coaster ride takes its toll, though. No matter how much you enjoy the thrill of the ride, eventually you want the ride to end—you want your feet back on the safe, comfortable, familiar ground.

Part of the ecstasy associated with my job related to Nathan. Nathan was a handsome, charming, witty waiter who flirted outrageously with me at every opportunity, as did many of my male customers. For the first time in my life I felt both pretty *and* desirable. After having spent much of my life loving men who did not share my feelings, I *needed* to feel wanted. My tendency to love men who not only did not want my love but who also put me down at every opportunity was slowly destroying my happiness, my joie de vivre. Daryl, with his occasional passes, had managed to quell much of my self-confidence. Knowing that I had feelings for him, Daryl still made advances towards me and then apologized for having done so. I now see his behavior as cruel thanks to the wisdom that comes of age and very expensive antipsychotics.

I was both independent and needy at this time. I could live with or without friends. Thanks to my family's many moves, I was accustomed to being alone. And with my many interests and hobbies I was most proficient at filling in the friendless gaps as they arose. I did not *like* being alone—I wanted to have friends. I was, however, interested in making real friends only. Fly-by-night acquaintances never appealed to me.

Could I live as easily without a boyfriend? Sadly, at this juncture in my life I wanted a boyfriend badly. More specifically, I wanted to find my soulmate and live happily ever after. True love was what I wanted most out of life from as early on as I can remember. Like I said, at age 3 I had planned on marrying the little boy who lived down the street. To me, the sole purpose of life was to fall in love and marry. It did not occur to me that life's winding road could lead elsewhere. I did not and do not equate marriage with the loss of one's independence. I would marry, but I would remain true to myself. No matter how needy I may have been regarding men, I was always sufficiently independent that I did not change myself to please a man. I did not hide my intelligence, nor did I hide my musical abilities. I was always Janet. A man would have to take me as I was. In addition, I never dated a man for whom I did not possess real feelings. In the course of my life I have had two marriage proposals, but I refused both because I was not in love. I was not going to marry for the sake of being married, so my neediness never destroyed my independence.

Nathan, the waiter, had a girlfriend whom he neglected to mention at first. Had I been apprised of this information, I would never have allowed myself to develop feelings for him. I had already sailed on the ship of unrequited love with Daryl and, thanks to my newly found pride, was well on my way to throwing myself overboard when Nathan entered into my life.

The night I found out that Nathan was "torn" between his current girlfriend and me, I lost it. What little pride I possessed at this time disappeared. I went into a depression, an abyss, lower than any I had ever known. And I became outraged, angry, furious! That same night I went to a house party. Upon finding myself alone with Nathan, I reamed him out about his flirtatious behavior. I was screaming and crying (I could see Nathan was stunned and a little scared), but I could not stop. I yelled at him that he had no right to lead me on the way he had, that he had no right to hurt me as he had done. He tried to placate me with apologies, but I was not listening. I was completely lost in my sorrow, my pain. I wanted him to feel the pain that burned through my body, depleting me of my physical strength and rendering me slumped over on the living room floor. Like a child I sat on the floor hunched over, head in hands, crying, and rocking back and forth. To me, Nathan was no longer in the room. I was alone in my misery. And then, as quickly as you can switch on a light, I stood up, smiled brightly and apologized to Nathan for my getting "carried away." My about-face frightened him even more. I could see that. And I was mortified that I had behaved like a madwoman, but the damage was done.

I have pinpointed my manic depression as having started at this time because of this incident with Nathan, this loss of self-control. Screaming at someone, crying in front of someone—these actions were not part of my normal behavior. Why I blew up at Nathan and not Daryl, I do not know. Clearly, I was sick; unfortunately, I was the last one to figure that out. This episode with Nathan was a one-time-only thing, and almost instantly I was back to normal.

I thank God for my cocktail waitress job because it gave me back some pride, some sense of importance. Regardless of the episode with Nathan, at this time I felt good about myself in general. I remember my mom hating the fact that I was waitressing because she believed I was wasting my God-given talents and intelligence. I guess I did not realize how much I needed this job to feel worthwhile, and so I could not explain my love of the job to my mom.

I now realize pride is intrinsic: you give it to yourself. They say pride is one of the seven deadly sins, but I know from experience that the absence of pride is lethal. Without it, you are completely vulnerable, a target for those who live to use people. And users abound in this world.

After the Nathan incident, around the beginning of May, a waitress friend named Susie introduced me to her live-in boyfriend, Niles. She had told me a little about him. From her I had learned that Niles was an alcoholic whose only job was doing the lighting for a band. I interpreted this information to mean that he was living off of her. Whatever.

I met Niles and was smitten. I knew instantly that my feelings for Niles were stronger than any I might have had for Daryl, Nathan or any other man I had met. It was pure, true love. True love!

I could not believe my rotten luck.

Who am I trying to kid? Of course, I could believe my rotten luck. Now, good luck—that would be unbelievable!

I still had a hands-off policy regarding men who were already in relationships. I was ethical . . . and alone. And I was constantly fighting off Niles' advances. I even told Susie, in a roundabout way, that Niles was flirting with me and that I was not sure how to handle the situation. She laughed and told me not to worry about it, adding that Niles was "just being Niles." What I failed to disclose were Niles' protestations of love for me. Niles was frequenting the lounge almost nightly whether Susie was working or not. One night he pulled me into his lap and said, "Janet, I love you. You know I do."

I laughed and said, "Tell me that when you're sober, and I

might believe you."

But I did believe him. There was something about his eyes . . . but unable to forget about Susie, I got up and walked away.

One Friday evening in May, Susie had an impromptu party at her apartment after work. It must have been around 2:00 a.m. when the party started. In attendance were some of the wait staff from the lounge and their dates. There were some new faces, as well, but basically it was the usual crowd. We listened to music and had a few drinks. Again, the usual.

And then, somehow, Niles and I were alone. Everyone had left, including Susie. Immediately Niles moved closer to me on the couch and put his arm around me. I told him not to do so, but he protested that he loved me and only me. And I believed him. I could have just stayed there sitting on the couch with Niles for the rest of my life, and I would have been happy—dare I say "content." This combination of closeness and serenity is one that I have not experienced again . . . except with . . .

With Susie in mind, I half-heartedly pushed Niles away from me, uttering, "You live with Susie. She's my friend. This isn't right."

But Niles persisted in remaining close to me. I decided to go to the kitchen ostensibly to get us a couple of beers. I really had to get away from Niles before I did something unethical, wrong and possibly hurtful. Upon closing the refrigerator door, I turned around and found myself face to face with Niles. He put his hands around my waist, pulled me towards him and kissed me. I did not and could not stop him. The kiss felt right. I could not summon up any feelings of guilt at this moment. I loved Niles; that was that. Niles was, of course, Mr. Jones—Charlie, Lenny, Nick, Niles Jones.

Perhaps I should have suspected that something did not ring true about Niles. At work, Susie had often referred to Niles as "Keith," and at the time I had questioned her about her use of the two names.

"Niles is eccentric," she laughingly replied. "He likes to change his name . . . a lot."

"So what *is* his real name, then?" I asked.

"Keith. Keith Jones."

I was still in Niles' arms when my feelings of guilt quickly returned. I pushed Niles away from me once again, and we returned to the living room . . . to talk. Again I said, "You're living with Susie. You can't be with the two of us. When you know who you want to be with, then I'll listen to you."

Susie came back to the apartment as I was finishing my sentence. I figured it was time to go.

I did not see Niles again. I lost my job at the lounge at the end of May. I never understood why. My tips were always good, and I was popular with many of the customers. From what I could gather, someone had phoned in a complaint about my service, and the manager had chosen to believe the complaint. I cried when I lost my job because along with the job I lost my friends—and my hopes of seeing Niles again. Susie had told me that she would be leaving Edmonton in June to go to work in Banff, a mountain resort town in Alberta. Niles was supposed to be leaving with her.

Oh, by the way, whenever anyone asked how I was doing during this time, my reply was always the same: "I'm bored."

Chapter 14

I fell into a deep depression when I lost my waitress job, the kind of depression in which you just want to sleep your life away. Seeing Daryl was the only thing that could lift my spirits at this time. Even though the drive to Fort McMurray took about five hours, I made the trip regularly. Daryl visited me in Edmonton too, and . . . he began hinting that he might move to Edmonton in the near future.

My mom and dad—my whole family, really—had no idea how depressed I was. I was always changing my face, my attitude. My mom thought I had some sort of split personality. In a way, she was right. Happy Janet was ecstatic about life and its many possibilities; sad Janet just wanted to be dead and in Heaven.

I used to blame my parents for my misery. After all, they chose to have a child, to have me. I had no say in the matter, as do none of us. I remember saying to my mom, "Why did you have children? Who gave you the right to create life when all I am is miserable? *I wish I'd never been born.*"

My mom always responded, "Life is a gift from God. A *gift*. He loves you. You need to believe in Him and His plan for you."

Of course, her words fell upon deaf ears. Depression has a habit of rendering you deaf to any words or ideas that might actually do you some good. I mean, when you are in the abyss, some part of you wants to remain there because that is the easiest thing you can do.

I think, in my case, that I wanted to maintain my depression simply because I was so good at being depressed. Depression was familiar territory, and in an odd way remaining depressed showed stability, perhaps even control.

I was inspired just now. I like to think that when God talks, I shut up long enough to listen. And no, I'm not hearing voices. I just think any momentary brushes with genius I may experience come straight from God, the Big Guy—the really, really, really Big Guy. I'm too young to be wise and too wise to be young. Now where did that come from? Mania truly is an enigma.

When I came out of my depressed state in September 1987, I decided I needed a change. It seems that I have always needed changes in my life to feel happy or happier—changes within my control, that is. The negative changes, those forced upon me, typically have rendered me depressed. Anyway, in order to get on with life, I decided to try something new and completely different, to give myself a new direction. By this time I no longer thought a career in music a viable choice. I had already been in two bands that went nowhere, and I was far too nervous to play solo. Banking it was.

When I was a child, my Grandpa Ronnie used to say that I would make a great bank teller because, like him, I was "good at numbers." For whatever reasons, at this time his words came back to me, and I resolved to follow up on his advice. I telephoned every bank in my area of the city and was hired the same day by a small, friendly bank situated about ten minutes from my home by car. The bank hired me with the stipulation that I would have to learn the teller job within ten days, or they would have to let me go and hire someone with direct experience. Three days later, I knew the job cold. The girl who had trained me was going on maternity leave; I was therefore hired to be her replacement for the duration of her leave. Because I learned the job so quickly, she left after my fifth day in training.

I liked my bank job. It was mellow for the most part. I worked with a girl my age and we got along fine, but we were not friends. We did not socialize.

I took pride in my work. My cash balanced to the penny every day because of my overwhelming need to be perfect. Whenever things slowed down during the day, I would double- and triple-check my work, ensuring that my cash balanced at all times. I became obsessive in my desire to balance. If I were out even a penny, I would search for my mistake until I found it.

In order to be perfect, one must make mistakes. The inability to err would be a flaw since perfectionism includes the ability to do anything, to make a "perfect" mistake. (Janet's convoluted logic.)

I became so enthused with my job that I spent my weekends studying courses, which I got from my employer, to learn more about banking. My objective was to become a loans officer, but a promotion to a supervisory position would have pleased me. I enjoyed the banking environment; it suited me. Indeed, I found myself looking forward to Mondays. As with my cocktail waitress job, work became my life. I no longer frequented nightclubs or pubs. I lived for my job.

Can you feel the cynicism?

Yea, though I workethed mine ass off, I was kickethed in the teeth once again.

In February 1988 the girl who had taken a maternity leave returned, and I was left with the offer of a part-time position that I declined. Needless to say, I was angry and hurt. The other full-time teller—the girl with whom I had worked for the past six months—made errors daily, but I was the one whose hours were being reduced. "Seniority," they said. "Fear," I determined. I was too good at my job and thus posed a threat to those above me. I closed my account at the bank thinking, "Fuck you."

My, oh my. A lady doesn't talk that way—unless the lady is completely, utterly, totally pissed off!

Anger is not always a negative thing. Sometimes anger is the only thing that can lift me out of depression. Anger almost always follows sorrow, but this anger is simply a feeling and not anger directed towards someone.

Think I'll regret myself again
Or I'll protect my right to sin
> *Tired and haggard*
> *But I will face the fight—on my own*
> *Anger moves me*
> *To pick myself up off the ground*
I heard you say "It's just my way"
Lead me on.

Excerpt from song "Drink" © 1994, J. M. Knudsen

Rather than permit myself to go into yet another deep depression, I immediately chose to take on a new project. I enrolled in the Certified General Accountant program, which offered accounting courses by correspondence. After having received the highest grade in Canada on my first exam, I quit the program. The one thing I learned from taking this course was that I did not want to be an accountant. Oh well.

In March 1988 I applied for and accepted an office clerk job with the federal government. Basically, the job entailed typing correspondence. The hours and pay were great compared to what I had been earning in the years following my stint as an insulator, and being well paid was my only consideration now. I had learned the hard way that loyalty to a company and hard work do not pay. In addition, I had discovered that every time I found a job I truly loved, I lost the job. No, from now on my only job-related concern would be the amount on my paycheck. Job satisfaction now varied directly with my income.

One April weekend, my youngest sister Tammy and I drove to Fort McMurray to visit our friends. I went to see Daryl, of course, and the weekend was typical of my visits with Daryl. We went dancing at a nightclub, we ate out, and we talked a lot. The drive home to Edmonton, however, was not typical. Far from it.

Tammy and I left Fort McMurray around 8:00 p.m. Sunday night. We had a five-hour drive ahead of us on a long, lonesome highway. As usual, we listened to music while driving. Light snow began to fall after about an hour on the road. I was not too worried. I was used to winter driving. With still an hour of driving to go before arriving back in Edmonton, I had an eerie feeling—a feeling that something was not right with our choice of music. I turned to Tammy and said, "We should listen to something else. Put in a different tape."

But Tammy wanted to hear the next song, the very song with which I felt at odds. My mind was telling me that if I heard that song, which contained the lyric "goddamn," something bad would happen. The song came on, and when the lyric in question rang out, the car hit black ice and went careening off the highway into a ditch. I cannot express how lucky we were. The left side of the highway was heavily wooded. Had we slid off the road in that direction, we surely would have been killed. Instead, we slid into the ditch on the right side of the highway where a blanket of soft, newly fallen snow cushioned us into a slow, safe stop. Although neither one of us was wearing a seat belt, we did not suffer so much as even a bruise. We were, however, in a ditch in the middle of nowhere. Literally. We were at least an hour away from any town in any direction. It was 11:00 p.m., and by now the falling snow had become a blizzard.

I did not know what to do. I activated the car's hazard lights, and Tammy and I walked to the edge of the highway . . . and waited.

I believe in miracles.

Within five minutes of our crashing, a couple of truck drivers came along and stopped when they saw us. Their truck was equipped with a winch, and they managed to pull my car out of the ditch and back onto the highway quickly and easily. They waited to see if my car worked and if it looked like we could make it home. They even offered to drive ahead of us slowly for a while to make sure that we would be OK. I do not think I believed in good Samaritans until this day.

It was 1:30 a.m. when Tammy and I arrived home. Interestingly, my parents had had bad feelings about us, about our safety, and they were still awake waiting for us when we walked into the house.

Retelling the story of the car crash brings to mind another near-death experience.

In Montreal when I was 8 years old, my class from school went on a day trip to the mountains to see where and how maple syrup was made. Upon arriving at the mountains around 10:00 a.m., we were split up into groups of six children to two adults so that we could go hiking for a few hours. My group was determined to reach the top of the mountain; accordingly, we went off on our own to seek the path to the top. And we did reach the top.

What a feeling! I felt so close to the blue sky that I stood up on my tiptoes and reached upward as high as my little arms could reach in an effort to touch the sky, to touch Heaven. Thinking about this moment, I understand why people want to climb Mount Everest.

> *Look up high, watch the planes as they fly by*
> *As a child, I thought that I could hitch a ride*
> > *But I say, "Hey, now, now*
> > *It doesn't matter anyhow"*
> > *And I think, "Hey, my, my*
> *Does the dreamer have to die*
> *Does the dreamer have to die."*

Excerpt from song "Hey, Mon Dieu" © 1991, J. M. Knudsen

It was getting late. All of the groups were supposed to meet up at the sugar shack around 1:00 p.m. It was already 12:30 p.m. when my group arrived at the mountain's pinnacle, and we knew that it would take us well over an hour to hike down the mountain on the same path that we had taken when climbing it. So the group leaders scouted the mountain and spotted what looked to be the fastest route to the bottom.

We hiked downward until we came to a snow-covered slope. We figured we could slide down this incline and save a lot of time in so doing. The adult male in our group, Chris, went down first. Next, a boy from the group slid down. I followed. What we could not see from where we had been standing was that the slope ended abruptly, becoming a cliff. Chris had managed to grab and hold on to a tree trunk just before he reached the cliff's edge. He shouted to us not to come down, but it was too late. The boy and I were already sliding downward. Somehow, Chris managed to pull both of us off the slope and to safety. I remember standing near the edge of the cliff, horrified! I kept staring at the drop. I did not scream; I did not cry. The silence was deafening.

Chris said, "Janet. Janet! You're OK. You're OK!"

I did not respond. Chris's voice was distant, far away from me, just a vague sound. I kept looking for the bottom of the cliff—I could not *see* the bottom. The drop was enormous.

"Janet!" Chris grabbed my arms and shook me. "Janet!" he shouted, looking me in the eye.

"What?" My voice was soft, almost inaudible.

"We're OK. We're all OK. Let's walk back up, now."

He held my hand and the three of us slowly worked our way back up to where the rest of the group was waiting.

In view of this catastrophe, the group leaders decided we would climb down the mountain using the same path we had originally taken. We were late getting back to the meeting place. I think it was around 2:30 p.m. when we plodded into the sugar shack, tired, exhausted. One of the teachers in charge of the day trip gave us hell for going off alone. I *really* did not need to be scolded at this moment. I thought the teacher in question was utterly devoid of compassion! This teacher wanted to punish our group by not letting us eat the pancakes, sausage and maple syrup lunches we had been promised.

My teacher went off with Chris and the other group leader to find out what had happened. She called me over to this group and asked, "Why did you go off alone?"

My response: "What's the point of climbing a mountain if you're not going to go to the top?"

Laughter. My teacher laughed so hard she almost cried. She went over to the other two teachers in charge of this outing to discuss the situation. She argued that we did nothing wrong, at least not intentionally. And so my group had lunch. The food was cold, but we had our lunches. I do not think a pancake ever tasted so good!

Chapter 15

Following the car accident, things stayed pretty much the same. I continued to work for the federal government and was given a special assignment that I loved. I was happy with my job and with my coworkers.

"Happy with my job."

Again, this phrase does not bode well for me. Alas and alack and bloody hell!

The special assignment ended after a couple of months, and I earned a letter of commendation for my efforts. I was disenchanted upon returning to my original typist position. Indeed, I could no longer stand it! Bored silly I was. The only thrill I had when typing correspondence was correcting grammatical errors. The only thing that kept me going was the hope of being promoted.

And I deserved a promotion. I had over two years of university education and was well versed in three languages: English, French and Spanish. Having been educated in Quebec, I knew French well. And while working at this government job, I quickly taught myself the basics of Spanish at home in my spare time. One day at work I was asked to translate for some newly arrived Spanish-speaking immigrants and was more than happy to do so. I loved being able to put my knowledge to good use.

I think the word "quota" must be Latin for "You're fucked."

Thanks to the quotas in place at this time, I was passed over for a promotion. I did not fall into the right category according to the quota criteria. The promotion went to someone far less skilled than me, rendering me completely disillusioned with my job. Accordingly, when my six-month term was up at the end of July 1988, I chose not to renew my contract. You might say that I "quota'd" them right back!

While still working for the federal government, I began to go out to nightclubs again. Only now I sported a new look. A more daring look. My hair was cut short and dyed black, and I habitually wore sexy, formfitting, black Lycra miniskirts or mini-dresses teamed with silver jewelry and silver chain-link belts. My black-on-black phase was in full bloom. When working as a cocktail waitress, I had often been told that I had nice legs. At long last, I had developed the confidence required to show them off. For far too long I had been a homebody. The loss of my waitress job had curtailed my desire to go out to clubs and bars. Now, at 23, I was finally starting to live again.

My youngest sister Tammy was in attendance at an arts-oriented high school and had adopted the Goth look. Upon meeting Wanda and me, John—Tammy's longtime boyfriend—asked us to join Tammy and him for a night out. He thought it was absurd that Wanda and I were always home alone. I do not know why, but at 23 I felt I was too old for the nightclub scene. John assured me that many people in my age group went out to the clubs.

So, one Friday evening in July the four of us headed out to a local diner/club to see a blues band. The Diner, as I call it, had a '50s motif that included pink walls, black and white floor tiles, mini-jukeboxes at each booth and photos of famous movie stars from that time period. And the best burgers in town. Instantly, I felt completely at home here. Most clubs made me tense; not so The Diner. I knew right away that I would return to this place again and again.

The band that night, Wild Horse, was excellent. I made it a point to remember their name so that I could see them again in future. They played covers of The Doors and Jimi Hendrix, and they played well. As a musician, I tend to be critical when it comes to live music. I expect to see accomplished players when I go to a club and pay my cover charge. Wild Horse easily lived up to my expectations.

That night at The Diner I had fun! Finally! Fun *without* Daryl, fun *without* a date. Just me having fun. And this was new to me. For so long I had believed that I needed a boyfriend, or some male companion, in order to enjoy myself when going out on the town. Daryl felt like a boyfriend in many respects, but he was just a friend, albeit my best friend.

Wanda and I returned to The Diner the following Thursday that July to see a solo act. I walked into The Diner, dressed to kill, and ordered a beer. I was still a two-beer kind of girl, three if I knew I was in control. To be in control at all times was and is as essential to me as breathing. My weight obsession is a perfect example of my need for absolute control over my body; remaining sober exemplifies my need for absolute control over my mind.

Around 9:00 p.m. a young man with long black hair—decked out in black jeans, a white shirt and black cowboy boots—came on stage. Just one look and I thought to myself, "He's the man of my dreams. He's the one I've been looking for. It's him!"

He sang Bob Dylan and Neil Young songs for the most part, but he captured my heart when he sang his own songs. He was brilliant. His words were thoughtful, romantic and often profound. And his melodies . . . I wanted to write melodies like his. I was in love. Totally in love. I smiled so much that my face ached, but I could not stop smiling. All I could think was that I had to meet him, but how? I lacked the courage to go up to him and to talk to him directly. Never having been lucky in love, I was a coward when it came to meeting men.

Thank You God!

To my surprise and joy, he came over to our table and introduced himself. His name was Keith Jones. I had no recollection of having met him in the past. This was our first meeting as far as I knew.

When he talked to me, he looked deep into my eyes. No man had ever talked to me this way. He compelled me to return his look, to look into *his* eyes. I had long been in the habit of looking at people's mouths when they spoke—perhaps I feared what I might see in their eyes. But here I was staring deep into Keith's eyes, unable to look away, unwilling to break the spell. He spoke, but I was not really focused on his words, their meaning. My head was swirling, my smile becoming brighter and brighter, his words lingering in the air like music . . .

"Janet!" Wanda spoke and broke the spell.

"What?" I responded angrily, for she had interrupted my bliss.

"He asked you what your name is."

Returning my glance to Keith, I blurted out, "Janet. My name is Janet."

Still looking into my eyes, Keith said, "Janet. That's a beautiful name."

I thought he was crazy. My name was plain, dull, ordinary. I asked him his name.

"Keith Jones," he replied.

"It suits you—I like that name."

He laughed and said, "I've always thought my name was boring. Are you sure Keith Jones is a good name for a musician?"

"Yes, why not?" My response was immediate. "I don't understand why musicians change their names, anyway. They should be proud of what they do. They *should* take the credit for their songs. If I wrote a song, I would use my name."

"Are you a musician?" His look was curious, probing.

"I play the guitar . . . and I try to sing. But I can't write songs. I think people who can write their own songs are geniuses. I wish I could . . ."

"You've never written a song? Not even one?"

I was somewhat startled by his intensity. I responded, "No . . . oh, yes. I did write a song once when I lived in Fort McMurray, but I don't like it. I just don't have what it takes. It's too country, and I want to write rock." I had completely forgotten about my song *Trusting Child,* a metal song, because I deemed it more a poem than a song.

"I guess you don't like my music." His voice was soft.

Totally aghast, I looked at him and said, "Your songs are the best original songs I've ever heard! You have catchy melodies and the words are great. I love your songs. I really do!" All I could think was that I blew it. I loved this guy and had managed to screw things up in the space of five minutes. How stupid could I be?

Keith looked back at the stage for a second. He then looked me in the eye—he always looked me in the eye—and said, "Thank you. I'll keep that in mind."

He left our table to return to the stage and sang *Tangled Up In Blue* by Bob Dylan. Watching him and listening to him sing, I felt like the song was about me, that he was singing for me and me alone. I wanted this night to go on forever, but Wanda had other plans. She was tired and wanted to leave. I had no choice but to go with her. It was around midnight when we headed home.

I have often wondered why I have negative thoughts about Wanda when I am in a paranoid state. I believe the bad thoughts probably stem from this one night, the night she interrupted and then ended my bliss. I now realize that I was being unfair to her. She had no idea that I loved Keith. He and I were meeting for the first time, after all. And Wanda was tired even before we left the house to go out that night. I had agreed with her that we would go to The Diner and leave around 11:00 p.m. Despite having to work the next day, she remained with me at The Diner until midnight. I love Wanda, and I feel terrible for ever having thought negatively of her.

I told Tammy about having seen Keith Jones that Thursday, and she asked, "Keith Jones? Isn't he the leader of The Smoking Guns?"

I replied that I had no idea whether he was in a band, that he had not mentioned a band.

Tammy said, "I'm sure he's the singer for The Guns. They're playing at The Diner, Saturday. You should go."

And so I planned to do just that.

Daryl, true to his word, moved to Edmonton on Friday, July 29, 1988, the day before The Guns' gig at The Diner. He was fortunate in that he had obtained a job transfer that enabled him to relocate without loss or interruption of income. And I was happy to have my friend living near me once again, but one thing had changed in the dynamics of our relationship: I no longer viewed Daryl romantically.

Keith now held that special place in my heart.

Groan . . . how cliché, how corny and, oh, so trite. I'm a romantic fool. Sh! Don't tell anyone. It's a secret.

Daryl stayed at my family's house that Friday, and he and I went apartment hunting first thing Saturday morning. We found an apartment near my house in no time, and I helped Daryl move into his new place. My parents gave him an old couch and a loveseat. Since he was comfortably settled in early that same afternoon, I gave him a tour of the city to help him learn his way around.

Daryl moved to Edmonton primarily to start up his own blues band. I wanted to believe he was moving here for me, but I knew better. For Daryl, being in a band in Fort McMurray was a dead-end situation. He hoped to be signed to a record label and could not possibly achieve this goal with his band being based in such a small town, so he made the big move after his bass player set up residence in Edmonton.

The band would practice at the bass player's house. I was supposed to play keyboards—again with the keyboards. Blues was not my cup of tea any more than metal had been when I formed my first band in Fort McMurray. However, I wanted desperately to be in a band, so I acquiesced . . . to the style of music. I put my foot down when it came to my playing keyboards only. With the arrival of Keith into my life, the need to please Daryl in all things had vanished.

Yes, my attitude changed that quickly. Virgos are known to be mercurial, and I am the "mercurial girl."

I informed Daryl that I would play keyboards solely as a secondary instrument. Either I would be the rhythm guitarist or I would not join the band. Having recently purchased a dark gray electric guitar, I naturally wanted to play it! Period!

Daryl looked baffled. I had never really argued with him before, never asserted myself. At long last, I was growing up. I was realizing that my opinions and feelings did matter. And I now had a notion in the back of my mind that Daryl was manipulative, that he was playing *me* in a way. This notion, new to me, was one that I did not like. But I could not get this thought out of my mind.

I asked Daryl if he would like to go with me to The Diner that same night to see The Smoking Guns.

"Oh, I was hoping we could go to a movie and relax." He had that persuasive, cajoling tone in his voice that I had heard so many times, the "you agree with me" tone.

But for the first time, I did not agree. Not at all.

"I'm going to go see The Guns. I've never seen them before, and I heard they're good. Tammy told me." Thus, my foot hath met the ground.

Again, Daryl looked baffled.

"I guess I'll go, but if they suck, I'm leaving," he muttered.

"You do what you want. I plan on staying for the whole gig."

Was this me talking? I did not say that . . .

That night I wore a ruffled black miniskirt, a skintight black tank top and a pink bolero jacket. I wanted Keith to notice me. I picked up Daryl and we drove to the club. To my surprise and distaste, Daryl noticed me in a way that I had never seen before. He eyed me lasciviously; I felt uncomfortable. Even when Daryl had made advances towards me in the past, his face had always been expressionless. The lust now evident on his face was unsettling. I mean, Daryl had once told me that he felt I was "not feminine," a remark that never left me.

We arrived at The Diner around 9:00 p.m. and ordered a jug of draft. Unlike me, Daryl was a drinker. There was no sign of Keith. For a moment I thought that Tammy was wrong, that Keith's band would not be playing this night.

At 9:30 p.m. Keith strolled into The Diner, glanced over at Daryl and me, and then went back outside. It was a beautiful, warm, sunny evening. In Edmonton the sun shines until late at night in the summertime, as late as 11:00 p.m., I think.

Belatedly, I realized that Keith might think Daryl was my date, and I found myself wondering how to mend this situation. Keith helped to mend it for me. He went around The Diner from table to table to collect the two-dollar cover charge. When he reached our table, I said, "Hi Keith. This is a friend of mine from Fort McMurray."

"Friend?" Keith spoke the word emphatically.

"Yes. Daryl and I have been friends for years. Daryl's

girlfriend is in Fort McMurray right now, but she might move here soon."

Problem solved.

Keith smiled brightly and said, "Enjoy the show."

I could not help but notice the look of disgust he shot Daryl; indeed, that look made me feel closer to Keith than ever before.

The gig was great! The music was a fast, lively mix of country, rock and punk that made me want to dance. The Diner, however, was not really a dance club. Since it was too small to have a dance floor, I bobbed and swayed to the music while seated. God, I was happy!

Daryl hated the band. He wanted to leave after the second song. But with my newfound sense of importance I said, "Fine. You go. I'm staying."

"Poor" Daryl looked somewhat sheepish and said, "O . . . K . . . I'll stay."

I really did not give a rat's ass what Daryl wanted. It was *my* turn. It was time for me to have my say. I had been meek and agreeable for so long that I had forgotten what it was like to "do what I do," to follow my desires. Take me as I am or do not take me at all—that was my attitude when I was a child, a healthy attitude that got lost somewhere along the way while I was growing up.

After the first set, Keith came to my table and asked how I was enjoying the gig.

"It's great!" I replied. "I love your music. The only thing is I wish I could dance in here. I'll have to see you when you play at a place with a dance floor."

"We don't often get gigs in bigger clubs. But I'll try." With that, he grinned and walked away.

Daryl was noticeably silent that night. Whatever. I was happy. Hap, hap, happy! We stayed until the end of the gig, and I left looking forward to the next. As I was leaving, Keith said, "I'll be here on Thursday again. Come if you want."

"Yes, I'll be here."

But I did not go. Daryl's friend Jack arrived in town that Thursday afternoon . . .

Chapter 16

Jack was a buddy of Daryl's from Fort McMurray, where they had worked together for a while. Jack was not my type. Not at all.

Daryl and I picked up Jack at the bus station Thursday, August 4, 1988. Jack had been on an extended European vacation and was now returning to Canada, to Fort McMurray. Edmonton was supposed to be a stop on his way home.

I had planned to go to Keith's gig at The Diner that evening, but I could not find anyone to accompany me. Daryl and Jack were not interested in seeing Keith, and my sisters were unavailable. Instead, I ended up at Daryl's apartment where we were just going to have a drink or two and talk.

Jack was at the apartment when I arrived. Daryl had offered to put him up for the weekend or longer, if needed. The three of us spent the evening looking at photographs of Jack's European holiday. God, I was bored. I thought to myself, "It's Thursday night, I wanted to see Keith, and instead I'm stuck here looking at pictures of some stranger's holiday. Whoopedy-fucking-ding-dong."

Around 10:00 p.m. I left. Jack did not want me to go; indeed, he did his best to persuade me to stay. And knowing that he was attracted to me, I was all the more anxious to leave. I mean, if I were attracted to either of these two men, it was Daryl who interested me. I had had a thing for Daryl for a long time, but I already knew that what I had felt for him had fizzled out and died, Keith or no Keith. For sure, Keith was now first in my mind and in my heart, and I viewed Daryl as a friend and nothing more. Regardless, Jack I did not like— not one iota. I did not like his looks, nor did I care for his personality. I felt extremely uncomfortable when near him.

The following evening Jack was still at Daryl's place. I learned that Jack was entertaining the idea of remaining in Edmonton. The plan was that he and Daryl would share an apartment. I really was not happy to hear that.

The three of us went to The Diner around 9:00 p.m. that Friday night in my car. We were supposed to be celebrating Jack's birthday. The band Wild Horse was playing when we arrived, that blues band I liked so much. I had two mugs of draft while at The Diner, and I basically ignored my companions. I watched the band intently while Jack and Daryl got hammered. These two seemed far more interested in each other than they were in me. Fine. Whatever.

Since I was the chauffeur that night, I stayed sober. Staying sober was my norm, anyway. When the band finished their gig—and some time before that, truth be told—I was ready to go home. Jack and Daryl were not. Daryl persuaded me to go to an after-hours Latin nightclub situated across the street from The Diner. Although I voiced my protestations, ultimately I agreed to "one drink and home."

The Latin club was located in a dark, dingy basement. But it had a dance floor, which raised my spirits a little. I did love to dance, after all, and I knew Daryl would dance with me if asked.

A waitress came over to our table to take our order. She informed us that the bar served highballs only, no beer. Remaining sober was foremost in my mind, so I thought it best I have a soft drink.

Daryl argued with me: "Come on, Janet," he said. "You're sober and we're celebrating Jack's birthday. Let me buy you *one* drink."

Daryl was correct about my being sober. I was sober . . . and miserable. Jack's presence had ruined the evening as far as I was concerned. I just wanted to be alone with my friend Daryl. Oh well.

I gave in and ordered a vodka and seven, figuring it could not hurt.

Daryl went with the waitress to the bar. I think he needed matches. He was still absent from our table when the waitress returned with our drinks. I scanned the club looking for him, but he was nowhere to be found. "The bathroom," I surmised. "He must be in the bathroom."

And so I found myself alone with Jack. Ugh! When I thanked our waitress in Spanish, she looked completely astonished. She then asked me if I spoke Spanish.

"*Un poco*, a little," I replied, and she and I carried on conversing in Spanish until Daryl, at long last, returned to our table.

And then I noticed. Daryl was drunk, perhaps stoned. His eyes were glazed and he teetered when he walked. I had seen him drunk before, but never like this. I was worried about him, very worried.

Jack, on the other hand, was the picture of sobriety; and my logic told me something was wrong with this picture. Both Jack and Daryl had been drinking at The Diner. I had watched as they matched each other drink for drink. So why was Daryl out of it? I did not understand.

When Daryl took his seat at our table, I said, "Daryl, I want to go home *now*."

Daryl slurred, "No . . . let's dance."

Long in the habit of giving in to Daryl, I agreed to a dance. Right away I could see that he was having difficulties with his balance, so after two dances I insisted we return to our table. We sat there, quietly sipping our drinks. When Jack left to go to the bathroom, I informed Daryl that I was not happy and that I did not appreciate having to spend my evening with Jack.

"What's the problem?" Daryl asked. "I don't get you. Jack's a good guy."

"To you!" I retorted.

Upon returning to our table, Jack asked me to dance. At this point I was so angry with Daryl that I figured, "Why not?"

As I was dancing, the room started to spin. It felt, to me, like the floor was rising and sinking. I could hardly stand. It was a concentrated effort not to fall down. I remember Jack smiling at me, saying what a good dancer I was. My gaze returned to the dance floor. I had to stare at my feet to ensure that they did in fact meet the floor.

After one dance I excused myself to go to the bathroom. I was sad. Studying my facial expression in the bathroom mirror, I realized I was sad. And my head would not stop spinning. Something was wrong with me—I knew that much—but I could not pinpoint the source of my dizziness. I resolved to go back to our table and call it a night. Arriving at our table, I said, "I'm going *now*!"

Again, Daryl had disappeared. I told Jack to find Daryl immediately, or they could find their own way home. Within minutes I saw Jack practically carrying Daryl out of the bathroom and over to the staircase where I was waiting. Together we helped carry Daryl up the stairs and across the street to where my car was parked.

Jack said, "Janet, I don't think you're sober. You'd better let me drive."

"No!" My tone was forceful, emphatic. "I've had two and a half drinks tonight. I can drive. You're the one who's been drinking all night. Not me!" And I kept my car keys.

Once more, Jack tried to argue over who should drive. He had managed to infuriate me by now. I said, "Take a cab if you want. It's *my* car. I decide who drives it."

"All right. You win," he conceded. "Just drive safely."

"I always drive safely!" I responded. Who did he think he was? Who the fuck was he to give me orders?

Daryl's apartment was situated about five minutes away from the club by car. When we arrived at the apartment building, Jack asked for my assistance in getting Daryl up to his third-floor apartment, insisting that he could not handle Daryl on his own. Jack, a stocky, muscle-bound sort, could not manage to carry little Daryl up three flights of stairs? An alarm went off in the back of my mind, but I was feeling too disoriented to pay it heed. All I knew was that Daryl was my best friend and that he needed my help.

Somehow we managed to get Daryl up the stairs and into his bedroom. Lying on the floor, Daryl moaned and vomited up blood. I was scared. I wanted to call 9-1-1 because I thought Daryl might be dying. But Jack, his tone conciliatory, dissuaded me from doing so, saying, "No, don't be silly. Daryl is just drunk."

I stared down at Daryl. He continued to moan, and again he coughed up blood. I reiterated that we should phone 9-1-1.

At this point, Jack "took control." He found a pail in which Daryl could vomit. He placed a towel on the floor beside Daryl so that the bloody vomit would not ruin the carpets.

"I'm going home. You look after Daryl." I was exhausted, so very tired.

"Don't go yet," Jack pleaded. "At least wait 'til we know if Daryl is OK. Just stay for ten minutes, that's all. I'll get you a drink."

"No thank you. I don't want a drink. I'm tired. I'm going." All I wanted was to leave, to go home to my comfortable bed and to forget this night.

"But aren't you worried about Daryl? You know you are." Jack's tone was persuasive.

"Yes," I said, "but . . ."

"Ten minutes. Come on. Just ten minutes." Jack walked me into the living room and then went into the kitchen to get me what was supposed to be a soft drink—I had insisted that I did not want alcohol.

With one sip of my drink, I knew . . . "This tastes like gin. I told you I didn't want a drink." I was angry, but by now fatigue had taken over. Indeed, I felt physically drained.

"One gin," Jack coaxed me. "I hardly put any in there," he said, as he sat down beside me on the couch.

And then he put his arm around me. I did not, could not, move. The room was spinning as it had at the Latin club, only now I was seated. In a matter of seconds, Jack undressed me and was trying to . . . I had no strength. My arms felt like two dead weights. I tried to push him off of me, but it was like trying to move a brick wall. He kept saying, "I love you. You're so sexy . . . so sexy . . ."

"No!" My voice sounded far away from me. "I don't . . . No! Stop!"

I remember staring at the lamp that my parents had given Daryl as I was being raped on the couch that my parents had given Daryl. Jack tried to push my legs apart. I fought him as much as I could in my weakened state. "No! Stop!" I repeated over and over, but my pleas seemed to spur him on all the more. "No! Stop!" My voice faint, fearful.

My eyes remained on the lamp throughout the rape. In focusing on the light, I felt as though my soul had left my body. Jack continued his assault, but I was no longer there. I was in the light now, aware of the rape but separated from it at the same time. And then I began to pray:

"Hail Mary, full of grace, the Lord is with thee . . ." And the rape ended. Right away, it ended.

I am being explicit in detailing the rape because at the time it happened, I was too embarrassed—too ashamed!—to talk about it at all. Women have been taught from early on that it is unfeminine or rude or crude to discuss the vagina, and therefore women are afraid to say that they have been raped. A lady does not talk about such things, right? To make matters worse, women have been taught to think that rape is their own fault and that they have somehow invited the rape to occur. The end result is that women suffer in silence. They bury the rape in the deepest recesses of their minds and hope never to think on it again.

I looked at Jack. His face was pure evil, his lust evident. And then he noticed the blood . . . lots of blood . . . everywhere blood . . . *my* blood.

I saw that Jack was covered in blood from head to toe. I then realized that I, too, was covered in blood. The couch was soaked with my blood. The room looked like a murder scene, only I did not die.

I arose and made my way to the bathroom, leaving a bloody path where I had walked. I was not really conscious of my actions— some other part of my mind had taken charge. Without thinking, I stepped into the bathtub and turned on the shower to wash the blood away. I was crying now. I could not stop the torrent of tears any more than I could stop the bleeding. You know the scene in Alfred Hitchcock's *Psycho*? I felt like I was living it. I remained in the bathroom for at least ten minutes, waiting for the vaginal bleeding to stop. But it did not stop. I waited and waited, but the bleeding would not stop. Jack was knocking on the bathroom door.

"I wish the knocking would stop. I wish he'd go away!" I thought.

The knocking continued. I did not know what to do. What is the correct course of action when something like this happens? What is one supposed to do?

Jack was now pounding into the door in an effort to break the door down. Quickly, I grabbed a towel and covered myself. I then opened the door, thinking, "Daryl can't afford to replace the door if Jack breaks it."

I let Jack "help me" to the loveseat. I know I got dressed . . .

Jack asked me if I was still bleeding.

"Yes," I replied, still crying, "but it'll stop. I'm going now."

"No!" Jack was shouting. Why was he shouting? "You can't leave while you're bleeding. Just wait awhile."

"I'm supposed to wait. Yes, I probably should wait," I thought to myself.

I waited.

Jack put his arm around me as if to comfort me. I could not *think*. In my mind I repeated, "I need to think. I need to think. Let me think."

I was still crying . . . and then I stopped. Just like that, I stopped. I looked at Jack, smiled and said, "I really have to go now."

His bewilderment was obvious. I was smiling. I knew I had to keep smiling.

Daryl came out of his bedroom.

"He's up. Oh good. I'm glad he's OK," I thought.

After looking at the blood-soaked couch, at Jack and at me, Daryl said, "It looks like you two had fun." And he *grinned*. The little asshole was grinning.

"I have to go now," I uttered. "I'm glad you're better. I have to go now."

And I got up off the loveseat and walked towards the door. Jack followed. He followed me down the three flights of stairs and out to my car. He said, "I think we'd better go to the hospital."

I gave him my car keys. He "sped" me to the nearest hospital and carried me into the emergency room in his arms. How heroic.

At the hospital I was given an ID bracelet dated August 6, 1988, and was led to a cubicle to await a physician. By now I had been bleeding profusely for at least two hours. I was crying again. A nurse came in, looked at my tear-soaked face and asked sternly, "Why are you crying? Does it hurt?" She handed me a feminine napkin.

"No," I replied.

"Then stop being such a baby. You don't need to cry if it doesn't hurt."

So I did what I was told—instantly I stopped crying.

After another ten minutes had gone by, a doctor came into the cubicle. He performed a vaginal examination. Grinning, he looked up from my vagina to my face and said, "It looks like you and your boyfriend had fun."

"Fun?!" The word exploded in my brain. To the doctor I retorted, "He is *not* my boyfriend!"

"Whatever," said the doctor. "It looks like he cut you. Was he wearing a ring?"

"I don't know. He's not my boyfriend. I don't know him. He's my friend's friend."

This shithead of a doctor then said, "I'm sure it's nothing. The bleeding will stop by itself. You can go." With that, he left the cubicle.

I was still wearing my miniskirt from the night before, and I believe this doctor formed his own negative opinion of me on sight. I left the cubicle and returned to the waiting area. Jack was there.

"The doctor said I can go home now," I stated.

Just outside of the hospital, Jack said, "I'll take a bus home. You go. I'll be fine."

So I got into my '83 Capri and drove home. And I really do not know how I made it home. My head was swimming. I remember that I was trying to think. I needed to *think*. I had to figure out what to do. I did not want my parents or my sisters to know what had happened. I could not and would not let them know. I had to keep it a secret . . . *I HAD TO THINK!*

I returned home around 8:00 a.m. Saturday morning. My older sister Wanda and I still lived with our parents at this time. I went directly to my bedroom, lay down and waited for the bleeding to stop. And waited.

My mom came into my room and asked me if everything was OK. I told her that I was fine, that I just needed some sleep. I put on my smile, knowing that I could fake happiness and *believing* that I had to fake it. Nobody was allowed to know what had happened. Nobody! My mom checked in on me again and told me that she and my dad were going out. I told her to go, that I was fine.

Around 10:00 a.m. I was still waiting for the bleeding to stop. I had been lying in my bed for two hours, waiting. The phone rang.

"Janet!" my sister Julie yelled out. "Janet! It's Daryl."

Picking up the telephone in my room, I said, "Hi."

"Hi. I'm just calling to see how you are. Jack is pretty worried about you." Daryl sounded well.

"I'm fine," I responded. "Tell him not to worry. I'll be OK."

"Jack wants to talk to you," Daryl informed me.

Without pause I said, "I don't want to talk to him," and I hung up.

I then called out to Julie, asking her to come to my room. "Julie," I said feebly, "I need to go to the hospital."

Julie was not really surprised. She had stayed at the house at my parents' request to ensure that I was all right.

"Julie," I said, "I need for you to drive me. I've been bleeding and I don't think I should drive." Julie had never driven a car before, but I insisted, saying, "I'm with you. It'll be fine."

She then asked me about the bleeding.

Quickly I responded, "Oh, it's a woman's problem. I put in a tampon wrong or something. Anyway, I'm not worried, but I really do need to go to the hospital now."

Accordingly, Julie drove me back to the same hospital I had visited earlier that morning. I was still wearing the ID bracelet from my first visit. The admitting nurse rushed me to a cubicle and a doctor was summoned immediately. A different doctor—not the one I had seen earlier. Right away this new physician asked me what had happened.

"I don't know," I answered. "I've been bleeding for about

four hours. I was here before, but the other doctor sent me home."

Examining me, the doctor asked, "Janet, were you raped? Did this guy force you . . ."

"No," I replied swiftly, "I don't think so."

"But someone did this to you. There's a cut on the hymen. That's why you're bleeding." His concern for me was evident on his face and in his voice.

Again I said, "I don't know."

The doctor, changing focus, asked, "Do you know the name of the physician you saw earlier?" He paused. "Who sent you home?"

I gave him a description of that doctor; I could not remember his name.

"You need stitches," he said. And he proceeded to close up the cut.

"Janet," he continued, "listen to me. If you were raped, you need to tell me. I can't help you if you won't talk about it. Was it rape? Was it someone you know? Is that why you won't tell me what happened? *Was it someone you know?"*

"I don't know. It doesn't matter. I'm not bleeding anymore, right?"

He nodded.

"Well, I'll go home now. Thank you." And I went home . . . with my secret.

Do you know what really broke my heart? After my night with Tristan, my first, I promised myself that the next time I gave myself to a man, I would have to be in love with that man. I was going to wait until I found my soulmate—the man with whom I would spend my eternity. Jack took this away from me. He raped me. My martial arts training could not help me. I had been slipped a drug while at the Latin nightclub, a drug that rendered me defenseless.

Jack raped my body. And Daryl raped my soul. Between them, I was broken.

Janet Knudsen

Tired Soldier

If it's more, I want it
If it's less, it's mine
Can you guess—maybe not
The hurt so hard to find

When I was a young girl
Innocence was lost
Hard to tell—maybe not
The hurt, it had to cost
Oh, the memories—searing flames
The hurt, it had no name
And me, I'm not to blame

Oh, the tired soldier
Chains across his face
Fighting for me—yeah, I think
The soldier's full of grace

If it's more, I have it
If it's less, it's gone
Can you guess—maybe so
It's you and we're our own

Can you hear me calling out your name
Can you feel me falling out of shame
Can you see me losing all my pain
Can't you hear me calling out your name.

Song "Tired Soldier" © *1994, J. M. Knudsen*

About one week after the rape, I went to a clinic—not to the hospital where I had gone when I was raped—to make sure that I was not pregnant and to check for sexually transmitted diseases. I was prompted to go by a nightmare. In the nightmare I was pregnant and hiding in my bedroom closet. There I remained for the entire pregnancy because I was ashamed and thought everyone would think I was stupid and irresponsible.

The medical examination took longer than expected. I remember the doctor calling in a nurse and saying something about having to "clean the area" where the cut was located.

My focus was not really on the doctor. As with the rape, I felt separated from my body, like I was watching from above. One thought rolled over and over in my mind: "I can't be pregnant. Please, God, don't let me be pregnant." And I was not pregnant, was I?

The doctor performed a D & C. I had no clue what a D & C was at the time or for a long time afterwards. Lately, I have learned that it is a scraping of the uterine lining. But all I knew back then was that a local anesthetic had been administered and that the doctor had worked on me for about five minutes, maybe longer. As I said, I was out of it.

This doctor's visit played a major part in my first and subsequent breakdowns. While delusional, I came upon the notion that an abortion had been performed on me without my consent. I knew that the doctor at the clinic had done something requiring an anesthetic, and in my mind that something was an abortion. As much as I did not want to be pregnant, I would never have consented to an abortion. Any baby of mine would have been loved without question or reservation.

My five-year descent into madness began with the rape. I concede that I was manic depressive prior to the rape; but paranoia, delusions and voices were new territory. As far as I am concerned, my mental collapse began with the rape and culminated in my being sent to the hospital psychiatric ward in August 1993.

Bitter, sad irony. About three weeks after the rape, I was offered a temp assignment with the Canadian Mental Health Association (CMHA). I accepted this five-day position immediately. I needed something—anything—that would occupy my mind. I was doing my best to forget the rape and to carry on as though it had never happened. My attitude at work was positive, upbeat, cheerful. I simply refused to think about the rape, to think about the blood . . . I had to live in the now and I *had* to look happy. My mask with its fake smile was impenetrable. Indeed, my boss remarked on how nice it was to be around someone with such a happy outlook on life. Mission accomplished.

Jack sent me a bouquet of red roses on my first day at the CMHA office. He was still attempting to woo me (over the telephone—I did not want to see him) and to apologize for the night in which he got "carried away." Fuck him! I let the fucking flowers die, die, die. I abhor the color red. If Jack had known me at all, he would never have sent me *red* roses.

That felt good. My anger is vented. I did not realize how much anger I still have towards Jack. If God forgives Jack, so do I. Forgiving, however, is not the same as forgetting.

I saw Daryl that same week. We were having our first band practice at the bass player's house. Although I was in a room with four other people, I was not there. To me, it felt like I was alone with my new, dark gray guitar—that it was just me and my guitar in this room. And that felt right.

Somehow Jack, who had come to the band practice with Daryl (Jack was not in the band), had it in his head that he was my boyfriend. Immediately I corrected him. Looking him in the eye, I said, "Sorry, Jack. I don't mean to hurt you, but I like Daryl."

I said "sorry" . . . to Jack!

When I now spoke to either Jack or Daryl, I made eye contact, daring them to meet my gaze. My face was stone cold, no fake smile, just a marble statue. Daryl noticed the change; that he had noticed was evident on his face.

Upon leaving the house, I got into my car and cried. I absolutely refused to cry in front of either Jack or Daryl. I started my car. Looking at the road ahead, I thought, "If I were to go fast enough, I could crash into that fence and die."

I remained parked in front of the house for a while, the car's engine running. I was smoking a cigarette . . . and pondering suicide. This was the first time that I truly considered taking my own life. Admittedly, I had given the subject some thought over the years, but I had always shrugged off this defeatist notion quickly. Borrowing a line from Scarlett O'Hara, I would muse, "I'll think about that tomorrow." And with each tomorrow, the suicidal thoughts would be gone. I *did* want to live and to achieve my dreams. Most of all, I wanted to find my soulmate, to love and be loved in return.

"Keith Jones." Still parked outside the house, I pictured Keith Jones in my mind. And with his smiling face firmly embedded in my thoughts and in my heart, I drove home.

If I killed myself, I wouldn't get to have another cigarette— now that's a perverse irony. Thank God I have a sense of humor!

This first band practice was my last. When Daryl called me to ask me to the next practice, I said, "Sorry, Daryl, but it [the bass player's house] is just too far from my house. Either you find a new place to practice, or I'm out." I could not help but add, "I don't like Jack being around all the time. If you like him so much, then *you* hang around him. I'm sure the two of you will be happy together!" And I hung up.

Daryl called me back later that day to apologize. He asked me to go to The Diner with him one more time. He then informed me that his girlfriend from Fort McMurray would be joining us. I told Daryl that I would go but that I would get my own table. I had no desire to be a fifth wheel.

Dressing sexier than ever before, I went to The Diner that night—and I now had attitude. After getting a lust-filled look from Daryl, I thought, "Good, you little shit! Now you want me, now you can't have me."

Daryl and Jack left Edmonton at the end of October 1988. They may have been players in The Game, the mind game that began so long ago with Sherry's murder.

Me, I started to go out on the club scene now and then. Basic black. Silver accessories. Happy expression. I had become the porcelain doll.

Chapter 17

I do not know why, but I remained in touch with Daryl even after he had moved back to Fort McMurray. My head refused to accept that he might have been in on the rape. Such betrayal was not possible, or so I thought. But my feelings for him had changed dramatically: there was no attraction, no desire. No longer did I journey to Fort McMurray. Daryl had to come to me. I know he noticed the change in my attitude towards him, as he phoned and visited me less and less. In fact, he never again stayed overnight at my house—my parents' house—following the rape. Our visits petered out to lunch meetings when he would stop in Edmonton en route to Calgary, Alberta, to visit his infant son. Ultimately, I told him that if these quickie lunches were the extent of our relationship, I wanted out. Acquaintances and half-assed friendships are a waste of my time. The last time I saw Daryl was just after Wanda and I had moved into our own apartment. He stayed over for one night. I never bothered with him again except to say that our friendship was finished.

At home after the rape I did my best to appear chipper. A lot of people around me at the time remarked on how nice it was to see me smiling for a change. My fake smile . . . I practiced smiling in mirrors all the time to make sure that my smile looked right. I also studied my reflection as it appeared without the mask. The misery was evident. In studying my reflection, I perfected my fake smile. Although my sadness then was overwhelming, I succeeded in keeping my sorrow—and its source—my secret.

The makeup I wore, a part of the mask, was always the same: blue-red lipstick, red rouge, dark blue eyeshadow and black eyeliner. The only time I can tolerate the color red is when it is a makeup color. I am not sure why. With my naturally ashen skin and blue-black hair, the "doll" look was complete. Seeing the character of "The Joker" in the movie *Batman* years later, I remember thinking that The Joker's face was a grotesque version of mine. This thought unnerved me, as I had worn that face for so long.

Following the CMHA assignment, I was offered and accepted a temp job with a lawyer. In my three days with this lawyer I completely overhauled his filing system. My constant need to be organized helped to get my mind off of my troubles, I guess. Usually. But by the third day of the assignment I told the lawyer that I would have to leave. The stress of the job was wearing me down, and I had to maintain my mask. I had to.

I was unemployed from November 1988 to March 1989. I slept on the sofa in front of the television day in and day out. On the rare occasions that I ventured out into the world, I donned the happy face. Over time, wearing my fake smile became as natural as smoking—I mean, breathing.

OK. This subject depresses me, so I made a sad attempt at humor just now. Don't feel bad if you want to laugh. I laugh all the time. It keeps me healthy.

My mom knew that it was not like me to do nothing. I told her it was "just a phase." I believed I would snap out of it sooner or later because that was my way.

Acceptance

What is life?
It's the edge of death
What is death?
It is peace and serenity
It's a longing
What is the longing?
It's the ability to—to
          be accepted for what you are
Your peace
Your serenity
Your longing

Poem "Acceptance" © 1994, J. M. Knudsen

During my phases I habitually pondered God, life and death. And thank God I always came to the conclusion that love does heal all wounds, even if the only love you know comes from Him.

In December 1988 Tammy's boyfriend John came over for dinner. Tammy, my youngest sister, was always naturally happy and always had a boyfriend. I deemed her my polar opposite. Indeed, I wanted so badly to be like her that it was her face I studied when perfecting my mask.

I refused to get out of bed that day. I had resolved to remain in bed until . . . whenever. John came into my room to talk to me, to give me a boost. He insisted that I was nice and pretty and that I should go out more. He felt certain I would make new friends if only I were out on the scene. John even offered to introduce me to his crowd.

I remained in bed, mulling over John's words. And then I perked up. "John is right," I thought. "I need to go out. I *will* go out."

John and Tammy asked me to go to The Diner with them that same December. The Alley Boys played that night, a band that I loved instantly. Their wonderful combination of '60s music and originals made me a fan. John knew the guys in the band socially and introduced me to them. They were nice and friendly, and I socialized with them from time to time afterwards.

When the gig ended around midnight, John invited me to a party at his place. Not having been to a house party since my cocktail waitressing days, I was thrilled. Finally I would meet new people.

The house from hell.

Upon arriving at John's place, I could hardly believe what I saw. Everyone was Goth. The furnishings were dilapidated, ready for the dump; the floors being used as ashtrays. And the place was wall-to-wall people. "Pretentious," I thought. "How very pretentious these people are."

John shared this Hell House with three other men: Hank, Jerry and Bud. Bud, whom I had previously met and liked, was John's best friend. My feelings regarding Hank and Jerry, however, were another story. I could not fathom how these two 25-year-old men could live in such squalor with nothing to their names. I thought it unnatural, strange, especially given that both Hank and Jerry were from upper-middle-class families. That these two had adopted the alternative lifestyle—Goth clothing, psychedelic drugs and living off the system—was obvious. Talking to them, I learned that they had no real plans for the future. Again, strange.

John and Bud I could understand. They were teenagers living out their wild days. But Hank and Jerry I did not get, nor did I want to. Indeed, they frightened me for reasons I could not quite understand. John told me that they were "harmless" and that they were "true punk rockers." My feeling was that they were pretentious, irresponsible shitheads. The "shithead" label stems from Hank's having made a crude joke about Jesus that I found utterly offensive.

The Game that started with the baseball murder of so long ago continued here at this house party. As usual, I did not recognize people from that time, from the murder. In 1990 I recalled that Hank and Jerry were the two students from The Asylum who had continually tried to get me to slip up and say that I had seen Sherry's murder. If you recall, I mentioned that there were three SOBs who constantly taunted me about Sherry back then. The third, Lars, was not at this party; but I eventually met up with him, too.

I left the party almost as soon as I got there. I did not belong. It was not my scene.

When Christmas arrived, I was severely depressed. As is the case with many people, Christmas always made me feel sadder than I already was. My poor mother. I told her annually that the only thing I wanted for Christmas was a boyfriend who loved me, which was, of course, the one gift she could not give me. I snubbed the presents I did get. My behavior was childish, rude, but I could not control myself or my feelings.

The promise of a new year, a new job and new friends kept me going. I did not go out on the scene again until March 1989. It was in March that I was hired to process paperwork for the provincial government. The pay was extremely good and helped to cheer me up a great deal. In my mind at the time, I needed either love or wealth to be happy or what passed for happiness. Finding this wonderful job inspired me to go out again, and it inspired me to pursue a dream that I had long ago abandoned. I now wanted to return to university and get my degree. I wanted to be a lawyer.

I phoned the local university and spoke directly to the Dean of Admissions for the business program. She invited me to meet with her so that she could see my school records and thereby advise me on my best course of action. Upon studying my records, she informed me that my credentials were more than adequate to gain immediate acceptance into the business program. Furthermore, she stated that she did not understand why I was not accepted years ago when I had first applied to this school. Instead of being angry, I decided to revel in my long-awaited acceptance and in the knowledge that I would get my degree at last. I would graduate with a degree in law by the time I turned 30, which was still young. I was excited and could hardly wait to return to school and renew my studies. Thankfully, September was not that far away.

Now employed, I began to think about getting out again and meeting new people. "The Diner," I thought. "I always liked The Diner." Accordingly, Wanda and I went to this favorite haunt the second Saturday in March. The blues band we liked, Wild Horse, was playing that night. We had a nice time, and we therefore decided to make it a point to see this band whenever they played in future.

It was not unusual for Wanda to accompany me when I went out on the town. We are only a year apart in age, our tastes in music are similar, and we have always gotten along well. We were and are best friends. Sisters and friends.

That night at The Diner I spotted a gig poster for Keith Jones hanging on the wall. The poster advertised that Keith would be playing a solo gig on the last Thursday in March for a two-dollar cover charge. I impressed upon Wanda my need to see Keith. Despite her disinterest in both him and his music (she preferred the blues), Wanda was a good sport and agreed to go with me to this gig.

We arrived at The Diner at 8:00 p.m. that Thursday, early enough for Wanda to have dinner prior to the gig. As an avowed "semi-anorexic," I allowed myself two fries, which I picked off of my sister's plate. By 9:00 p.m. only a handful of people were in attendance. I was baffled. Keith's music was so good that I expected a full house.

Keith took the stage at 9:30 p.m., singing a Bob Dylan song. I smiled when he played. I loved his music, his voice. He was the only person who could get a real smile out of me. The only one. To my joy, he came over to our table to talk to us while on his break. I remember him saying that he felt his musical career was being "sabotaged." He explained both the difficulties he was having in keeping a band together and the impossibility of getting gigs performing original music as opposed to cover songs. I commiserated with him, adding that I hoped he would succeed because I thought his original songs were brilliant. He then left our table but surprised us by sending us each a mug of draft.

I knew Keith Jones from the last few times we had met at The Diner, but I did not connect him to any of the times we had met prior to 1988. In other words, I did not realize that Keith Jones was Charlie, Lenny, Nick and Niles. I also knew that I was madly, totally, completely in love with him. He could do no wrong. And for my sanity's sake, I needed to love him. After the rape I was left with a need to be in love, a need to believe there was such a thing as a good, honest man. Because of his songs I decided Keith was that man. Now, I know that I was in love with a figment of my imagination. I loved who I imagined Keith to be and not necessarily who he really was.

Of note, I remembered everyone I met from 1988 onward. Prior to this time, when I bumped into people connected to Sherry's murder, they vanished from my conscious thought; but beginning in 1988 their faces, words and actions stayed with me. The "I don't know you" game would no longer work on me.

Meeting Keith gave me hope. And hope became love, and love became ecstasy. I was about to become completely manic—a mania over which I had no control, a prolonged ecstasy that proved both mentally and physically ruinous.

In April, a few weeks after Keith's gig, Wanda and I were invited to another party at the Hell House. Thinking I might meet people in my age group, I opted to go. Wanda declined. She did not like the alternative crowd and had no interest in getting to know them better. Even though I did not hold much promise for this outing, I was willing to give it one more try.

When I arrived at the party around 10:00 p.m., the place was a zoo. There were even more people in attendance at this party than had been present at the last one. Immediately, I scoured the living room in hopes of finding a familiar face. I succeeded. Keith Jones was there, and I became instantly happy and hopeful. Here was my chance! Here was my opportunity to talk to him and to get to know him on a more personal level. I was sufficiently realistic that I knew our conversations at The Diner might have been strictly business in his estimation. At this party there was no onus upon him to be nice to me.

I summoned up the nerve to walk over to where he was sitting and say "Hi."

Looking surprised, he said, "I didn't expect to see you here."

"I didn't expect to be here myself," I responded, "but my sister Tammy talked me into it." Staring into his blue, blue eyes, I added, "But I'm glad I came."

"So am I." His eyes locked onto mine.

There was an awkward silence before I blurted out, "Who's your favorite musician?"

"Neil Young, man."

"Neil Young? Really? I like some of his music, but I haven't really heard all that much of his stuff. Anyone else?"

"Bob Dylan, The Who . . . What about you? Who do you listen to?" He looked genuinely interested in my response.

"The Rolling Stones, Rod Stewart, The Pretenders, David Bowie . . . and Prince." These were the names that immediately came to mind. I continued, "I like lots of different kinds of music. Right now I'm really into U2. They have their own style. I think that's cool, you know, that they managed to come up with a new sound."

"I like U2," Keith agreed, "but The Rolling Stones and Rod Stewart? They're relics, man. How can you listen to them? You should listen to new music."

OK, he insulted my favorite musicians, but he was talking to me and I was happy.

Keith persisted, saying, "Those old guys had their day. You need to support new bands. New sounds. C'mon Janet. You're too young to be stuck in the past, man."

After briefly mulling over Keith's words, I said, "Well, Keith, those old relics are masters of music. The Rolling Stones are the richest band in the world because *everyone* likes them." Becoming more vehement, I added, "Keith Richards is my all-time favorite guitar player. I *want* to play like him! I'd be ecstatic if I could play like him!"

"Keith Richards," Mr. Jones said with disgust, "is an old, burnt-out has-been. Why do you like him?"

My answer was instantaneous: "Because Keith [Richards] loves guitar. He'd be playing the guitar even if he wasn't rich. You can tell he loves music. And, by the way, I'd rather be a 'has-been' than a 'never-was.' "

"Thank you." Keith's tone was icy.

"No!" I had to say something, anything, to vanquish his sudden coldness. "I didn't mean to insult you. I was truly referring to *myself.* You, I look up to. I wish I could write my own songs. I wish I had a good band. You're doing it! You're actually *trying* to get somewhere with your music. Me, I play by myself in my bedroom." I was talking too much. Shit! I always talked too much. Shifting gears, I said, "By the way, you remind me of Keith Richards when he was young."

"Great. So now I'm ugly too." Again his tone was cold.

"Are you kidding?" My bewilderment was evident both on my face and in my voice. "Keith Richards was really handsome when he was young. I think so. Even my mother thinks so."

At last, Mr. Jones smiled. "Thank you," his tone warm again.

Our conversation was interrupted at this point. A girl I did not recognize came over to where we were sitting and snarled, "Keith. Who's this?"

"Leah, Janet. Janet, Leah." Keith disinterestedly made the introductions.

Glaring at me with contempt, Leah said, "Excuse us. Keith is my boyfriend and we need to talk."

There was nothing to do but leave them. I was crushed. Keith had a girlfriend. I should have known. Although I wanted to go home right away, my pride would not permit it. I would not let it appear that I had attended this party solely to see Keith. I especially did not want Keith to know what I was feeling. So I looked around the room, and, upon spotting Tammy and her roommate Trish, I made my way over to them.

Trish struck up a conversation with me, saying, "I saw you talking to Keith Jones. Why on earth would you want to talk to him?"

"Because I like him," was my speedy reply.

"You *like* Keith Jones? Do you *know* him?" Trish continued her assault. "He's strange. He's always talking about a girl with long black hair. He's been looking for her for years. Everyone thinks he's weird."

"Long black hair," I rejoined. "I used to have long black hair when I was a waitress. But that was a long time ago, and I don't remember ever meeting him back then. Anyway, I've had short black hair the whole time I've known him."

I wished I were this girl with whom Keith was obsessed.

"But it doesn't matter anyhow," I continued. "He's dating that girl Leah, and she's got long black hair. Maybe she's the one he was talking about."

Looking at me in earnest, Trish declared, "Leah is a groupie.

She's always trying to get Keith to like her. He doesn't. She only dyed her hair black recently—like, a month ago. Don't worry about Leah. If he likes you, she won't stop him."

With these words, Trish renewed my sense of hope.

"If he is single, then I'm going to get him!"

Did I say that? It had never been like me to think this way. My rule was simple: if a man liked me, he would have to make the first move—he would have to come to me. Period.

The rape affected me in subtle ways as was evidenced by the changes in my thoughts and in my behavior. My resolution to pursue what or whom I wanted was new territory. Whereas even the smallest roadblock in the past would have stopped or impeded my progress, I now thought, "Fuck it. Try! If you lose, so what. At least you'll *know*."

Trish made one more statement: "If you really want Keith Jones, I'm sure you can get him. But I really don't know why you'd want him."

I was a bit miffed at Trish for insulting the object of my affection, but at the same time she made me feel like being with Keith was a real possibility and not some outrageous, unattainable fantasy. I left the party with a real smile on my face. Happy.

About a week later, Trish invited Wanda and me to a party being hosted by a member of The Alley Boys. There I met a woman named Bernadette who had a beautiful singing voice. Because so many musicians were present, a guitar was passed around. Those who could play, did . . . including me. Bernadette remarked that I was an excellent guitar player, that I was the best player there. So I asked her if she would be interested in playing a duet with me at The Diner's open stage night. She agreed.

Chapter 18

The next time I saw Keith was when his band played at The
Diner early in May 1989. Strangely, The Diner was packed. There
were more people than there were seats. Wanda and I had arrived
early enough to get a good table near the stage. For once, I was happy
that Wanda wanted to eat before the show.

The crowd included many faces from the Hell House parties.
I almost felt like I was becoming part of that crowd. Almost. The
band put on a good, lively show. Because I wanted badly to dance, I
asked Wanda if she would dance with me. Both in our mid-twenties,
we decided we were too old to care what others might think of us.
Accordingly, we found an empty spot near the stage and began to
dance. Within minutes everyone was dancing; and I then realized that
although people wanted to dance, they were afraid to be the first to do
so. Since I was no longer a frightened teenager, I resolved that I would
take the lead and be the first to dance. More importantly, I resolved to
do as I pleased regardless of what others might think of me—a new
attitude that stemmed from the rape.

Leaving The Diner that night, I felt utterly euphoric, on a new
high the likes of which I had never before known. That dancing gave
me joy is clear, but dancing combined with being in love rendered me
euphoric. This was a high from which I never wanted to come down.

I made up my mind to be happy and *stay* happy. In effect, I buried the rape in the deepest part of my subconscious, closed the door and locked it. It was as though it had *never* happened.

Are you, like, into crystals? (Valley girl accent.)

In 1989 the New Age movement was enjoying tremendous popularity, and my sister Wanda was one of its biggest fans. She bought tarot cards, astrology kits, crystals and rune stones. She learned how to read palms. Fortune-telling was her hobby, her thing. And although I never really bought into the New Age thinking, I did carry a pink rock with me everywhere I went. This pink crystal was supposed to attract love. I surmised that it could not hurt. After all, according to Wanda, all of the energies in the universe suggested that I was going to meet my true love at this time. I laughed at her prediction, but secretly I hoped she was right.

At work, things were great. I mastered my new job with the provincial government within a week and was quite pleased with the work itself. Though this may sound at odds with my personality, I preferred work that was simple and repetitive and that did not require much thought. I wanted to be able to daydream, to think about matters of importance to me . . . to think about Keith.

One of my coworkers hailed from Jamaica. I told her that I had visited that beautiful island and that I loved its silver jewelry. She astounded me one day at work by presenting me with several pieces of silver jewelry that included a charm bracelet and a bangle. I was floored. Although I immediately offered to pay her for the jewelry, she graciously declined. I faithfully wore the bangle from this day forward in the hopes that it would bring me luck. There was no reason for me to think the bangle was lucky. I just decided that it was.

Since I was single and had no real hopes of getting to know Mr. Jones better—he had not asked me for my phone number, nor had he said anything to imply that he might be interested in me—I went out on a date with John's friend Bud one evening that May. Tammy, John, Bud and I went to a popular, artsy café downtown. Tammy and John came along so that there would be no pressure on either Bud or me.

Bud was very cute and very nice, but he was also five years

younger than I, a fact I could not overlook. I felt more like an older sister to Bud than I did a viable love interest for him. The date, however, gave me a much needed ego boost, and I thoroughly enjoyed the evening.

Between Daryl and Jack, I had no self-esteem. They had hurt me in more ways than the obvious. The invisible hurts—no ego, no pride, no confidence and thinking I had only myself to blame—did the real damage to my psyche, my soul. For all my bravado (being the first to dance, for example), I was utterly devoid of confidence.

Tammy, who had moved into her own apartment at age 18, was heavily into the alternative scene. She now lived in an ultra-artsy, old building with cage elevators and beautiful hardwood floors. She shared this apartment with her longtime friend Trish, the girl with whom I had spoken at the last Hell House party. Although Tammy had adopted the Goth look, she did not share their mentality. Indeed, Tammy was what was referred to as a "poseur," meaning that she dressed the part but did not live it. Tammy's Goth phase was actually a rebellion against the preppy crowd whom she did not like at all. She found the Goths to be friendlier and more accepting. Being the new girl in school, this acceptance was important to her.

Unlike true Goths, true punkers, Tammy worked steadily from the moment she graduated high school onward. Her apartment was always clean and cared for. Many Goths were exploring witchcraft and Satanism. Tammy did not. Tammy's older boyfriend John was the true alternative, or Goth, in this relationship. Whereas Tammy went along with the crowd, never really aware of the negative aspects of the alternative scene, John knew exactly what he was doing.

Tammy and John split up in May 1989. Tammy met her now husband Ryan in July '89 and left the alternative scene completely.

While Tammy was making her exit from the scene, I was just beginning to hang out with the Goths, among them, Trish.

Right, then. It's time for some paranoid thinking. I wouldn't want you to think I was normal.

Years after meeting John, I wondered whether John had dated Tammy to target me. After all, it was John, and not Tammy, who convinced me to go to the alternative gigs and parties. Furthermore,

John made a pass at me following his breakup with Tammy that greatly confused me at the time.

They're out to get me! Or . . . maybe I'm out to get them? Now that's paranoia! I know I was attempting to be humorous just now, but this type of confused thinking plagued me when in the final days of my breakdown. This thinking exemplifies insanity in its truest, most horrific form.

Where was my head when I met the Goth crowd? I believed the Goths dressed up in black and silver for fun. Their strangely styled, oddly colored hairdos were just another part of the fun. My contention was that these vampires and zombies were indicating their musical preferences through their appearances. I had no idea that Satanism and the black arts ran rampant among this crowd. In my naiveté, I believed it was all about the music. Country music lovers wear cowboy hats, metalheads wear jeans and black T-shirts, and alternatives adopt a death-rocker look. It was all show . . . to me.

Was I Goth? No! At least I never considered myself as such. Yes, I wore black and silver and, yes, my hair was dyed black; but I was not trying to look like "walking death." And if I did, it was purely coincidental. I had been sporting black clothing since my days in Fort McMurray, and my blue-black hair was not cut into a punk style. If my face was white, it was naturally so. In addition, I did not adopt the layered clothing style the Goths so loved. My formfitting Lycra styles were in direct opposition to the Goth look. As far as I know, I was being me, Janet. Over the years, I have not changed all that much.

The last Friday in May 1989 I returned to my usual haunt, The Diner, to see The Smoking Guns once again. There were changes in the band's lineup, changes for the better. Certainly the band sounded more polished and more professional. I felt they were on the verge of greatness.

I wore my favorite black ruffled miniskirt, pink bolero top and black leather jacket that Friday night. The look, which had a definite Spanish flair, was everything. That I became obsessed with my wardrobe at this time is an understatement. I would change outfits as many as seven times a day because I felt each outfit had its own special "karma." And the karma had to be right.

This clothing obsession was clearly an offshoot of the mania that had now entered my life in full force. To me, my clothing and jewelry had tremendous meaning in the grander scheme of things. Not knowing exactly what that meaning was did not deter me. Looking right at all times was essential.

My ever-present silver chain necklace and cross seemed to ignite a rage on the scene. My cross was very special to me. I had found it at a flea market. This crooked, silver cross cried out to me! I knew it was mine, that I had to have it, that I was *supposed* to have it. Since virtually everyone on the scene sported all manner of crosses, I believed this crowd to be truly spiritual. I felt that I had at long last found my niche in this world.

Wanda accompanied me to The Diner that night. Even if she did not much care for the crowd or the band, she did like The Diner.

Wanda and I danced all night as The Guns made their assault. I danced nonstop. Literally. With a cigarette in hand and taking care to gravitate towards an ashtray when the ashes grew too long, I danced. I stopped only long enough to have a sip or two of my beer in between songs. I had to dance. As long as there was music, I had to dance.

OK. I know other people at the gig thought I was unusual, but I really did not give a damn. I was out to please me; my happiness was paramount.

*I just heard that the price of cigarettes is going up again. They **are** out to get me.*

Towards the end of the gig, around midnight, someone asked me if Wanda and I would like to go to a post-gig get-together at a downtown bar. After I consulted with Wanda, we agreed to go. Accordingly, Wanda and I drove downtown to the bar in question, The Watering Hole, and found a table for two. The place was packed, and for the life of me I could not figure out why. There was nothing to do at this bar but drink. There were no pub games or pool tables— just beer . . . and pizza. The Hole, as I affectionately refer to it, was actually a pizza restaurant with a lounge, but it was in the lounge where everyone hung out.

Keith was sitting at a nearby table with an entourage that I found daunting. I opted to stay at my table and wait. If Keith wanted to talk to me, he would have to come to me. He did.

"Hi Janet, Wanda," he offered. "It's nice to see you guys. How did you hear about this place?" He took up his position by my chair, leaning in towards us as he spoke.

"Someone at The Diner mentioned there was a party here, so we figured we'd check it out. It's cozy here, not too big," I prattled on nervously. "Do you hang out here much?" Good move, Janet. Turn the conversation over to him. Men like that.

"Yeah, it's my office, man."

I loved the way Keith used that word, "man." It was an expression that brought back my early childhood years, a time when I was happy.

"Your office?" I returned. "For the band, you mean?"

"Yeah, I do all of my business stuff here. And I drink. I practically live here, man."

Still nervous, I asked, "So do you have a job *other* than being in your band?"

"I'm the manager of my band," he replied. "That takes up a lot of my time. My mother used to manage us, but she was fucking useless . . ."

I was not sure how to interpret this remark about his mother. The venom in his tone was apparent.

". . . so now I'm in charge," he continued. "I get us gigs. I arrange the interviews."

"Wow! That's really cool!" I sounded like a silly, little girl. Making my tone more serious, more grown up, I added, "I guess someone has to be the leader of the band. I know. My bands never lasted long because nobody was in charge. It was a democracy, and that just doesn't work. It never works. Someone has to be the boss."

Keith now remarked that he was tired of standing, so I told him that he was welcome to sit on the arm of my chair. Then, gathering up every ounce of courage I possessed—having deeply weighed the pros and cons of the situation—I said, "I find you attractive."

I said it! I actually said it! My heart was racing, my body trembling. There was nowhere to go now but forward. "I *never* say that. But I just felt like I had to. I'm sorry, I probably shouldn't have said it. I . . ."

"You do?" Thankfully, Keith interrupted my rambling. "Really? Wow. I mean, thank you. I think you're really attractive too."

He thought I was attractive! Oh happy day!

"I . . . Thank you," was all I could manage in response.

"I have to go back to my table because my ass is getting sore from sitting here [on the arm of the chair]. We're all going to a party soon at Bud's house. Would you like to come?"

"I'll have to talk it over with Wanda, but probably . . . yes." Wanda or no Wanda, I was *going* to this party.

"Good. Please come." With that, he returned to his table.

Throughout our conversation Keith's "girlfriend," Leah, shot me looks to kill. But I decided not to worry about her. If she were indeed his girlfriend, that would be readily apparent at the party at Bud's house.

Although Wanda was ready to call it a night, it was around 1:00 a.m., I convinced her to accompany me to the party. "Just for an hour," I promised her. An hour would give Keith and me a chance to talk more. It would be enough time for me to discern, once and for all, whether he liked me romantically.

I was pleasantly surprised to discover that Bud and his roommates had moved to a new rented house. Hell House #2, as I dubbed it, was clean and nicely furnished. There were actual ashtrays available. Surprisingly, I did not feel at all out of place here.

After getting both of us a beer, Keith came over to me and asked me to join him on the couch. Sitting beside him, I was so nervous I could hardly think, let alone talk. Then Keith held my hand, and we sat there quietly watching the movie that was playing on the television. The silence between us was almost unbearable. Apart from asking me if I would like another beer, Keith said nothing. And since I was afraid of coming across as too needy or too interested, I remained silent as well. It was as if we had reached an impasse, neither of us willing to make the next gesture, the next move.

Wanda, who was soon fed up, told me she wanted to go. I knew I did not—not when Keith was holding my hand, not when my dreams were coming true. Breaking the impasse, I asked Keith if I could crash at his place. He quickly consented. I gave Wanda my car keys and told her that she would have to pick me up in the morning and that I would call and let her know where. Wanda then left.

It was all I could do to keep my eyes open that night. As much as I loved Keith, I had arisen at 6:00 a.m. that Friday and had put in a full day of work. Next, I had danced for three hours straight at The Guns' gig. When my watch read 4:00 a.m., I blurted out that we should go to Keith's place now. Insisting that he wanted to see the end of the movie, Keith left me with no choice but to wait. I remember watching the end of the movie, my eyes at half-mast, and thinking to myself, "Does he like me or not?" I had to know, so I used all of my will power to stay awake and see things through.

My entire life had been filled with silent crushes, and I was sick of it. Too many times I had played the good friend when what I truly desired was a romantic, loving relationship. "No more!" I thought. I would not repeat this guessing game with Keith. I would not put myself through that torment again. So awake I stayed.

Finally! The movie ended and Keith said that we should go. We walked from Bud's house to Keith's apartment. I do not know why, but I had assumed Keith owned a car. Whatever. Despite my being very cold as we walked, I was strangely happy. And oh, so nervous. As we neared his place, however, I found myself pondering whether or not I should call a cab and go home. Keith had remained silent during the walk, just as he had been at the house party. My head screamed, "What's going on? I don't get it! What's he doing? If he doesn't like me, he should say so. *I don't get it!*"

Then we arrived at his building. The warmth of the lobby was a relief; indeed, the warmth was inviting. The apartment building itself was an upper-middle-class complex, the sort of environment to which I was accustomed.

Once in the lobby, Keith took my hand in his rendering me completely reassured. We waited for the elevator for what seemed an eon. Finally, it descended to the lobby and we stepped into it, hand in hand. Now in the elevator, he kissed me. It was a soft, gentle kiss, the kind that promised love.

Am I writing a romance novel? Enough!

The rest of the evening stays between Keith and me.

I awoke the next day utterly, completely, totally in love with my Mr. Jones. I called my sister to come and get me, I went home, and I slept.

Chapter 19

But I did not sleep for long. Mania does not permit much rest.

There are many people who take all kinds of drugs to achieve a similar high to that which manics enjoy—or should I say, endure—not realizing or worrying about the destruction they do to their physical well-being. Would I remain manic if I could do so without suffering from the negative aspects of my manic episodes? In other words, if I could experience the energy and creativity that stem from mania without the negative side effects, would I choose mania? Having pondered this question at great length, I can only say that the answer currently eludes me.

While manic I wrote 82 songs in approximately a six-month time period. I wrote numerous poems, designed several sweaters. I delved into the meaning of life and came up with several God Theories, as I call them. And it was a brief manic relapse that inspired me to write this book. The rough draft was written in a mere 12 weeks.

My theory is that mania does not make you creative. Rather, I think mania ignites you to put your natural creativity into action. The "good" mania is a combination of extreme energy coupled with a super-positive attitude that allows you to accomplish a great deal in a very small time frame. But even the good mania is at best a fake happiness. For me, unfortunately, with the good comes the bad—the very, very bad that includes paranoia, delusions, visual hallucinations and voices. Because of the bad I now fear mania more than I enjoy it. Oddly, I am happiest when I am *not* ecstatic. Is that ever twisted! I guess what I am saying is that I would rather be on a natural high than on a manic high. One final note: I find my creativity has remained with me even now that I am normal, sane. It is as though the mania accessed a part of my brain to which I now have a free pass, manic or not.

That Saturday afternoon I went to Bernadette's apartment to practice a duet with her. She was the woman I had met at a party hosted by The Alley Boys. After practicing for about an hour, I hinted to Bernadette that I liked Keith. I will not quote her response, but the gist of it was that I should stay far away from him.

Naturally, I was miffed at her for denigrating my Keith. Although I say "my Keith," I knew that there was no relationship between us at this time. I left Bernadette's place in a bit of a huff but still prepared to perform with her the following evening.

I made my Edmonton debut on Sunday, May 28, 1989, at the diner I so loved. Sunday was open stage night, making The Diner the hip place to be. The liquor laws in effect at this time required that you buy food if you wanted to drink alcoholic beverages, so everyone ordered a plate of fries and a jug of draft. Hence The Diner's popularity.

I wore faded blue jeans, a white T-shirt with the sleeves rolled up and black sandals that night. This outfit was chosen in accordance with the energies of the universe . . . or I was trying to appear less Goth. Perhaps I chose not to wear black for the shock value. Based on the looks I received, people were indeed shocked, surprised. To them it must have seemed like seeing a nun out of her habit for the first time. I had my trusty pink rock in my left jeans' pocket, and I wore my lucky bangle. One does not mess with the universal flow— no bad karma for me, man. My sisters Wanda and Julie were in the audience, along with a friend of Julie's. I had my support team. I was ready.

I remember Keith went on stage first, playing his Ovation guitar. Ovations are the guitars with rounded backs that were made famous when Glen Campbell adopted them. Keith sang about seven songs, and then it was my turn. I had brought my six-string guitar with me, but my guitar lacked a pickup. To my surprise, Keith generously offered me the use of his Ovation, and I accepted.

Bernadette and I walked onto the stage. I was shaking so much I wondered whether I would be able to play the guitar at all. I was deathly afraid that I would drop my pick—like the world would come to an end if I dropped my stupid pick. But that was me, my nature. Anyway, Bernadette sang the first two songs while I accompanied her on the guitar. I sang the main melody of our third song with Bernadette singing harmony. Then my duet partner pulled the rug out from under me. She announced into the microphone, "Janet is going to sing '*Bobby McGee*' for you now." She then left me alone on the stage.

I was truly terrified to be alone, to play solo. However, the embarrassment I would feel were I to leave the stage outweighed my fear of making a fool of myself by singing alone. I strummed the intro to *Me and Bobby McGee*, a song that I had been playing since I was 12 years old, and nervously sang the opening line:

> *Busted flat in Baton Rouge, waitin' for a train*
> *And I was feelin' nearly faded as my jeans* . . . .

Excerpt from song "Me and Bobby McGee"
© 1969, Kris Kristofferson & Fred Foster
Combine Music Corp.

It is funny, interesting. I was extremely tired that night, but when I sang the part about the faded jeans, I perked up. I felt like *Me and Bobby McGee* was my song and that I was singing about me. There was a certain "oneness" about it that struck me loud and clear. My future thinking of "It's all one" stemmed from this song this night. Despite my relegating the oneness to being coincidence for quite some time, the notion of oneness remained with me forevermore.

Upon finishing the song, I was prepared to leave the stage. Through the applause I heard Bernadette shout out, "Sing *Crazy*."

"Oh God," I thought, "not that song." I was even more nervous. *Crazy* is a difficult song to sing well, and it is daunting to sing any song that Patsy Cline recorded in her day because you know you will automatically be compared to her. I hemmed and hawed, saying I did not really want to do another song and that Bernadette should be singing, when Keith startled me. He arose from his chair, stood on the floor directly facing the stage and me, and said, "Sing."

And with that one word, I sang *Crazy* like never before. Keith remained standing, just staring at me and listening to me sing. I felt both compelled and encouraged by his presence. But I avoided looking directly at him because I did not want anyone, including him, to know or guess that I had feelings for him. Since he had not phoned me after our night together, I figured that he was not interested in me. In addition, he was sitting at a table with Leah, leaving me with the thought that they must be together.

When I finished singing *Crazy*, the applause was tumultuous. I think I was in a state of shock by this point. I was running on adrenaline alone.

Keith said, "Do another one. You pick."

Thinking to myself, "Everyone likes Elvis," I sang my sole Elvis cover song, *One Night*. It had not occurred to me that Keith or anyone else would relate that song to him and me and *our* night together. The song went over very well. It was a '50s diner, after all.

Keith said, "More. Do more."

I was quickly running out of ideas. The only song that came to mind was *Dust in the Wind*, a song that required finger-picking as opposed to strumming. It was another song that I had learned when I was 12. Summoning up what little courage I possessed, I put my pick in my pocket and fingered the opening bars with their unmistakable melody . . . and everyone became silent. Keith, still standing, watched me intently. I was not really sure what to make of the look on his face. Did he like me? Did he hate me? I could not ascertain an answer to my questions.

Upon completion of this song, I said, "That's it. Thank you." And I left the stage.

I was shaking! The extreme fatigue, terror, excitement and

joy had taken their toll. It was an effort to walk the short distance from the stage to my table. If not for my mania, I probably would have collapsed then and there. Oh, but I was happy! Really, truly happy! At long last I had achieved my dream. I had played on stage, in public, in a big city, and I had been successful. People had applauded and encored me.

Scott, the lead vocalist for The Alley Boys, was in attendance this night. I had met Scott on several occasions and thought him good looking, but not as cute as Keith. Anyway, after playing, I went over to Scott's table to say "Hi" and to chat. Someone later told me that Keith looked upset when I was talking to Scott. I did not believe this news. In the two hours in which I had been at The Diner, Keith had made no effort to talk to me, to converse with me. My logic dictated that Leah was his girl and that I should forget about him. This was not high school, after all. I deemed all the "he said she said that they said" kind of talk childish. But admittedly, Keith was in my heart now, and I was prepared to give him a little more time.

The night I sang at The Diner, I chose my songs randomly, at least I thought I did. It did not occur to me that I sounded like I was singing about Keith and me until later that night when I was at home. The coincidence, the oneness, did occur to his friends, however, and was the catalyst that got The Game going in earnest once more.

I was in a fantastic mood when I went to work the next day. My mood was so good, in fact, that I decided to go with Wanda to The Watering Hole that night for a beer. Keith and his entourage were there when we arrived. Immediately Keith said, "Hello."

"Hi!" I responded. "I didn't expect to see you here."

"I told you. I live here." His tone was unreadable.

"Well, it's nice to see you anyway," I forged ahead. "Oh! I forgot to thank you last night for letting me borrow your guitar. That was really nice. I guess I'll have to get a pickup in mine . . ."

"You have it, you know," he said, interrupting my rambling.

"What?" I did not quite understand him.

"It! You have *it!*" He spoke the word with such finality.

"I don't know what you mean. Like star quality? No, I don't think so. I'm too nervous for that." Why did I always talk too much with this guy? Why did he make me so nervous? Damn!

"It's true. Everyone says so," Keith replied, gesturing towards his entourage. "We think you sing great. You may be the best singer in Edmonton."

"Sing? Me? God, that's weird. I mean, I play guitar. That's what I know how to do. I try to sing, but guitar is what I do." I meant what I said.

"You play guitar well," he continued. "Really well, man. But combined with your voice, you have *it*. You'll be a star." There was honesty and sadness in his voice. Not jealousy. Wistfulness.

"A star? No . . . I don't even have a band. I don't have songs. *You* may be a star one day. You have a chance," I said in earnest.

Keith looked away for a moment, then he turned his glance back to me and said, "I'm nobody. I'll always be nobody."

The conversation ended. He returned his attention towards his friends, and I went back to my table. I was sad. I knew I had hurt him terribly without meaning to do so, and I could not figure out how to fix it.

I intended to stay away from Keith the rest of the week. On Thursday night I met Bernadette at a downtown fast-food restaurant to discuss the possibility of performing with her again. She informed me that she was not really interested in playing on the scene, but she did encourage me to try. After she had finished eating—as a semi-anorexic, I never ate past 1:00 p.m.—she suggested we go to The Hole for a drink. Thinking Keith would be there and feeling certain that he did not want to see me, I told Bernadette it was a bad idea for me to go there.

Her reply: "Nonsense." With that, she convinced me to go.

When we arrived at The Hole, Bernadette was welcomed warmly. I got looks and felt stupid for having shown up . . . again. Keith and his crowd—he was perpetually attached to a crowd, an entourage—were talking about playing baseball on the weekend. They were debating whether Saturday or Sunday would be the best day to play.

Addressing Keith, Bernadette said, "I can come on Saturday. Hey! Do you need more players?"

"We always need more players, man." Keith avoided my gaze.

Bernadette continued, "Janet likes baseball. She should come. Right, Janet?"

Staring helplessly at Keith, I said, "Uh, yeah . . . I like baseball, but I'm no good at it. I don't think I should play . . ."

"Play. If you want to play, play." And so Keith gave me the go-ahead, and I smiled warmly at him in return. With the thought of work looming ahead the next day in my mind, I left the bar.

Bright and early Saturday morning I went out to buy a pair of white running shoes. Never having been sporty, I did not own anything suitable for baseball. In addition to the shoes, I found a cute white visor. Although I looked awful in baseball hats, the visor worked for me. I had succeeded in looking like a professional weekend wannabe athlete by the time I arrived at the park, and appearances were everything. Certainly, the other players shot strange looks my way, but I did not give a damn. *Keith* had invited me, the leader hath spoken, and that was that.

Immediately teams were chosen. Keith, as captain, did not choose me. Despite my disappointment, I understood. That he was under a lot of pressure from his friends and family when it came to me was becoming increasingly apparent. But not understanding why there was so much animosity towards me, I was greatly perturbed by this situation. I liked him and he liked me. What was the problem? And I do believe he cared for me at this time and for a long time afterward. For sure, it did not occur to me that his love for me might be a mind game. I loved Keith and thought he could do no wrong. His *friends* might have been playing games with my head, but not him!

After seven innings my team forfeited the game. To my surprise, Keith was really good at baseball and proved the best player among us. I say "to my surprise" because the vast majority of musicians I had met in my life were, like me, anti-sports. I was happy that his team won. I did not think our flimsy relationship could withstand another dent to his pride. I was happy just to be included. Not since my cocktail waitressing days had I been part of a group. The feeling that I belonged was exciting, and after the rape I wanted badly to belong.

The baseball game finished, everyone headed over to The Hole. At this juncture I must reiterate that although I was frequenting drinking establishments, I did so with a self-imposed two-beer limit. Only on rare occasion did I exceed this limit.

Now at The Hole, the girls sat together at one table, the boys at another. So I found myself sitting with the girls, who proved to be surprisingly friendly towards me. And after all the dirty looks they had given me, I was truly surprised. The girls were so affable, in fact, that I decided I must have misinterpreted those looks. Relaxing, I chatted with them for a while. But the notion that I was the newest member of a harem entered my mind, and I could not rid myself of this thought. To myself I thought, "Whatever. I like Keith. What the rest of them [the girls] do is their business."

Leah, Keith's supposed girlfriend, was especially nice to me. The discovery that we got along very well with each other baffled me. Then she said, "I slept with Keith last night . . ."

I did not hear the rest. My mind was whirling. "Did she say she slept with Keith? No, she couldn't have. No!"

And being manic, I began to interpret everything in a way that fit into my version of reality. In essence, I eventually believed that everyone was "speaking in code" and that it was up to me to decipher the truth from the lies. But in the beginning, I was rational about Keith and company. My early skepticism stemmed from the notion that this crowd did not truly like me, but rather that they wanted my support—and my money—at their gigs.

Because of my love for Keith, I interpreted Leah's having slept with him to be just that: sleep. Before I left The Hole, Leah and another girl, Yvette, gave me their phone numbers. Since I have always deemed the giving of a phone number a friendly gesture, I left feeling that I belonged. I left happy.

Chapter 20

I began to frequent The Hole more and more. On most occasions Wanda accompanied me, albeit reluctantly. On one such evening Wanda and I were invited to sit with Keith and a couple of the boys from his band. Yvette was there as well. We were all talking, getting to know each other. That Wanda and I hailed from Montreal came up early in the conversation. To my surprise, Peter, the drummer, mentioned that he too had been born and raised in Montreal. I said something *en français* to which both Peter and Keith immediately responded.

I never forgot this conversation. Never. Keith claimed to have been born and raised in Edmonton, Alberta, which is for the most part English speaking, yet he spoke fluent Quebec French. His French was *better* than mine. As the evening wore on, I noticed that Keith kept looking to borrow cigarettes from those of us who smoked. I am not greedy, but when it comes to my cigarettes, I put my foot down. I gave him one.

Then Keith ran out of beer money. He asked if anyone could lend him twenty dollars. When none of his friends agreed to the loan, I offered up the money. I did not want him to leave. And then I noticed Keith's bangles—he must have worn at least ten on each wrist. To my astonishment, one of his bangles was identical to the one I wore, the lucky bangle that had been given me by the Jamaican lady at work. In my mind, that our bangles matched went beyond coincidence. I thought to myself, "Keith and I are destined to be together. It's fate. It *is* all one."

Someone from Keith's crowd invited me to a house party the following weekend. I was on cloud nine. To be invited, included, was everything to me. Upon arriving at the house party, I scanned the living room looking for familiar faces . . . and looking for Keith. I spotted him sitting outside on the porch, alone. Gathering up what little courage I possessed, I went outside and sat down next to him. I wanted to talk; I wanted to know where I stood. In keeping with my new philosophy, I could not and would not harbor a silent crush on Keith or on any other man. I knew too well the misery of being in that position, so I asked Keith if he wanted "to get together again."

"No, sorry," he replied. "That was a one-time-only thing."

"OK," I said quietly. I then stood up and walked away from him with no intention of ever bothering him again. I had played my hand and lost, and I accepted my defeat. Yes, my heart was broken, but it would heal. There were other men. No longer would I waste my love on someone who did not return it. Oddly, between the rape and my night with Keith I now possessed a new, healthier view on men and relationships in general. My self-esteem went from being at an all-time low to as good as it had ever been.

In the house again, I sat on the living room sofa and pasted a smile on my face. That Keith had broken my heart was my business and mine alone. Within a couple of minutes Keith came inside and sat beside me. "Why?" I thought. "What's he doing?" I was understandably confused. He spoke first.

"I hope you understand the way things are," he offered. "I'm not trying to hurt your feelings. I like you. I really do *like* you. But that's all there is. I . . ."

"Fine!" I cut in, unwilling to listen to more of his conciliatory remarks. And with my eyes on his bangles, I asked, "Do you have my twenty bucks?"

"No. Not on me." His voice was low, his anger evident.

Still staring at his bangles, I said, "Well, give me your bangle as collateral on the loan." My anger matched his easily.

Handing over the bangle, Keith said, "Here. Keep it." The coolness in his tone was new to me, beyond anger.

"No," I returned, "I don't want to 'keep' it. I just want my twenty dollars. When do you think you'll have it?" I knew I had hit a nerve, and so I would not let it go. I wanted to hurt him. Why should I be the one who always hurt?

"In a couple of weeks," he replied. "I get paid in a couple of weeks, for sure."

"OK. Well, I'll see you then, but give me your [phone] number so I can make sure you have the money." I salted the wound. No one had ever angered me—or hurt me—this much.

"Fine." He then told me his phone number, adding, "Don't call before noon. I don't wake up until noon, man."

Getting up off the sofa, I announced, "This party is *boring*. I'm going to go dancing. See you." Was that my voice? I sounded so disinterested, so cold.

True to my word, I left the party with a girl from his crowd and headed to an alternative dance club downtown. I *wanted* to cry. I *wanted* to bawl my eyes out. Unwilling to give Keith the satisfaction of my being sad, however, I danced—for an hour straight. Then, at the girl's insistence, she and I headed back to the house party. Keith was not there when we returned. Leah told me that he had left the party shortly after I had made my exit. I found myself wondering what, if anything, that meant. Had he left because I had? To myself I thought, "Maybe he *does* like me. Maybe . . ." But not wanting to go that route, knowing that that kind of thinking almost always led to disappointment, I decided, "Whatever. I'll see him in a couple of weeks and get my money, and I won't bother with him anymore."

Once I returned home, I felt terrible. I had acted in anger, and I now felt disgusted with myself for having treated Keith so cruelly. I had not wanted to show distrust; I did not care about twenty lousy dollars. The truth was that I wanted to see the two bangles together, but I could not let Keith know my real motive. No way.

Following this fiasco, I did not know whether to socialize with Keith's crowd or not. Ultimately I decided, "Why not? They seem to like me." So I phoned Leah, and she asked me to meet her at The Hole that Friday.

Friday came, and I went to The Watering Hole where I found Leah seated at Keith's table. She motioned for me to join them. That I was uncomfortable is an understatement. Keith bailed me out, asking, "So Janet, are you coming to the baseball game tomorrow?"

I was baffled. Tongue-tied. I could not believe he was inviting me to the game—not after the collateral incident.

Well, laugh . . . God knows I'm laughing. The things I do for love . . .

I replied, "OK, if you want."

Looking me in the eye, he said, "No, Janet. If *you* want."

Wondering what was going on in his head, I agreed to go to the game.

Leah and I went from The Hole to a gig that Friday. We were out so late that I asked her if she would like to crash at my house. She did.

We arrived at the ballpark around noon the next day. Too exhausted to actually play the game, Leah and I sat on the sidelines, watched and cheered. And there I met a new girl, Doreen, who became my best friend in no time. There was no artifice about her. She, like me, was an outsider to the group.

After the game everyone headed over to The Hole. Once again I found myself at Keith's table. I was beginning to feel that there was, in the very least, some kind of friendship between him and me.

Leah remarked that I had the "perfect" family and a "perfect" house.

Keith asked, "So, Janet, which 'Brady' are you?"

His reference to *The Brady Bunch* irked me. I replied, "None. They're all too perfect."

"I don't know, Janet," he continued. "You're pretty perfect compared to us." And he gestured towards everyone else at the table.

For some reason, his remarks struck me as insulting. This guy who did not know me well was passing judgment on me *and* on my family. Calmly and oh so sweetly, I said, "Yeah, Keith, you're right. I'm perfect. And if I'm perfect and I'm hanging around you guys, you must be perfect, too."

So ended that conversation.

At this point I turned my attention towards Doreen. We chatted about school. I told her I would be starting at a local university in September. As she had attended that same university, she offered to show me around when the time came. I was nervous about finding my way around on such a large campus, so Doreen's offer afforded me tremendous relief.

You know what? I'm worried that I worry too much about worrying too much. God help me!

She and I agreed to meet at The Diner that night, where The Guns would be playing once again. By this time I was in the habit of going to all of their gigs. Keith's music was infectious. The feelings that lay between him and me were irrelevant. I loved his music, I loved dancing to his music, and I was not willing to forgo my euphoria so that he could feel more at ease.

Mania was now part of my daily life. I slept no more than five hours a night—on a good night. My thoughts were always racing, thinking that "something big" was in the works. I perpetually endeavored to connect the dots. I felt that my life was like a giant jigsaw puzzle and that I was finally fitting the puzzle pieces into their correct spaces. Indeed, the puzzle was nearing completion.

At the gig that Saturday night, Leah asked me whether I listened to Keith's songs.

"Yes," I replied. "Always."

"No!" Leah exclaimed. "I mean, do you *listen* to the songs?" Gesturing towards Keith, she repeated, "Listen!"

I listened.

And the clouds broke, and sunshine rained upon the land, while two birds of peace flew happily across the sky spreading their love and joy everywhere they flew . . . (Me, waxing poetic again.)

The words to Keith's songs were about me. Or, in the very least, the words to the song to which Leah had referred were about me. The lyrics described my actions, my words.

. . . and unicorns danced in the warm summer's mist . . .

(What a romantic fool am I.)

While singing, Keith's eyes remained upon me. Noticeably so. In fact, on this night and on many nights to follow, several people remarked to me that Keith was "obviously in love" with me. The relationship that I believed he and I shared was not entirely my fabrication, my delusion. I was being encouraged to love him.

Doreen, taking Wanda's place, began to accompany me to The Hole, to gigs and to house parties. She, too, encouraged my feelings for Keith: "He loves you. I can tell . . . everyone can tell." Smiling brightly, she added, "Listen to the words [to his songs]. Don't you see the way he looks at you? It's all about you."

Still skeptical, I told her I would believe he loved me when he said so . . . to my face . . . in *spoken* words. But Doreen insisted.

One incident changed me. One incident in particular convinced me that Doreen and Leah might be right. The three of us went together to yet another Smoking Guns gig in town. Doreen and Leah left to get drinks, leaving me alone on a bench in the lobby of the theater. Keith came over to talk to me. It was not what he said so much as what he did that turned the tide. He knelt at my feet, gazed upward towards my face and spoke to me. It felt like he and I were the only two people in the world.

"I see you're wearing the bangles," he said. "Do you know which one is mine?" His tone was gentle, no anger, no attitude.

"I . . . I'm not sure. I think it's this one," I replied, pointing to a bangle. "Anyway, Keith, I was just joking about collateral. Please take your bangle back. Please. . . and I'm sorry. I never intended to keep it."

Then Keith smiled at me and said, "Thank you." He left with his bangle.

That was the last time we had a moment alone together. After this tête-à-tête, at least one of his crowd was present at all times. The Game, I believe.

True to his word, Keith repaid the twenty-dollar loan within a few days of this meeting. I called him from work and arranged to meet with him at The Hole that evening to pick up my money. When I arrived at the bar, Keith was already there—along with two of the guys from his band. Immediately I thought, "He doesn't want to be alone with me."

Keith gave me my money right away. I felt so bad about the situation that I offered to buy a pizza for the group. I guess I wanted him to know it was not the money that mattered to me; it was the principle of the thing.

Yeah, there's a loan-related joke there. I love plays on words.

While awaiting the food, we chatted. Vic, the bass player, asked me whether I would rather have money, fame or power. (Where had I heard that before? My head was swimming.)

Peter, the drummer, asked me what my favorite color was. (Again, this question bothered me. It was such a commonplace query, yet I found it irksome. In fact, this entire scenario felt like déjà vu, but why?)

Keith . . . was *silent*. A venomous silence. I got the message.

I ate hurriedly, downed my beer and prepared to leave The Hole for what I thought would be the last time. During the course of my meal I had decided to leave Keith and his crowd for good. I reasoned that if he hated me, there was no point in trying to befriend his inner circle of friends. I could live without all of them as I had done before. The idea of being friendless did not scare me; I was used to being alone.

As I stood up to leave, Keith asked, "Are you coming to the gig on Thursday?"

OK, so now I was really screwed up. With his silence throughout the meal, had he not just made it clear that he did not want to know me? I replied, "I don't know. I have to work Friday."

His voice soft, he said, "Please come. And bring Wanda too."

He said "Please"!

With that one word, he broke my resolution to leave his crowd permanently. "OK," I said. "If you want me there, I'll come."

I left The Watering Hole, smiling. He had said "please." He did want me to stick around.

I went to the Thursday gig with Doreen. Wanda declined the invitation. My older sister did not like the alternative scene that included Keith and his friends. Even when I told her that Keith had specifically invited her to the gig, she did not care to go. Wanda thought everything to do with this crowd was "bullshit." Ultimately, Wanda was right.

After the gig, Keith invited a group of people to his apartment to watch movies. Even though I had to work the next day, I went to his apartment, happy to be included in the invitation. Surprisingly, Keith sat down beside me. We spoke quietly.

"Janet, do you ever wonder why you're here, man?"

"Yes," I replied, "all the time. I know God has a plan, but I have no idea where I fit in. I wish I did. I really wish I did."

"Have you ever been depressed? Really depressed?" He was genuinely interested in me.

"All my life." I spoke bluntly.

"But you look happy, man. Are you depressed right now?" Where was he going with these questions?

"Not right this minute, no. But I'm usually depressed . . . more often than not. I've just learned to live with it, is all. Why? Are you depressed?" I anxiously awaited his answer.

"Me?" he was thoughtful, continuing, "Sometimes. But not bad. I wouldn't kill myself like Frank [a friend] did. I'd never give up like that, man."

"I'm sorry about Frank. It must be hard to lose someone so close to you. I meant to say this at the time—I'm really sorry."

"Don't be," his voice now hard. "Frank was a loser. Suicide is for losers."

I had no response to that.

Keith broke the momentary silence, asking, "Have you ever thought about suicide? Would you ever kill yourself?"

Again I was dumbfounded. Taking time to gather my thoughts—and noting Keith's intent expression—I answered, "No, I don't think so. Whenever I think about suicide, I think, 'There's always tomorrow' and that keeps me going."

"But what if tomorrow sucks?" he pressed. "What if all your tomorrows suck? Then what?"

Another strange question. Regardless, I answered, "God did not intend for us to kill ourselves. If we believe in Him, then our lives will be what He wants for us. Sometimes we need to go through shit to appreciate the good. That's how I look at it."

With that, the conversation ended. I mulled over this strange inquisition many times, trying to determine the point of it. For one paranoid moment I thought that he was "feeling me out"; that is, I thought that he was trying to discern whether I would lose it, whether I would kill myself. But that thought vanished from my mind as quickly as it had come into it. I knew that line of thinking was paranoid, and I was *not* paranoid.

At the end of July 1989 I got my very first tattoo, which I designed myself. The design consisted of a blue G clef with musical notes shaped like hearts, and I had it tattooed on the side of my right ankle. I loved my tattoo! I had wanted one for a long time. Also around this time, I bought a blue heart of stone that I placed on the same chain as my cross. The cross placed over the heart represented my promise to myself to love Keith always, or at least as long as I wore this symbol. Remember, my clothing and jewelry were as one with the universe at all times.

Although The Smoking Guns were on the road for most of July, Doreen, Wanda and I continued to hang out at The Hole. We were bored much of the time, but then, there was nothing better to do.

Over the summer months I noticed Keith was becoming more and more distant. I wondered why he would not talk to me. He stared at me whenever I was near him. Doreen was certain he loved me . . .

One Saturday at the end of July, I invited Tom, the Confessor, to a barbecue at my parents' house where I still resided. He was noticeably both surprised and happy at the invitation. He came to the barbecue and enjoyed himself tremendously. As per the norm, my mom asked me to get my guitar and sing for everyone. I obliged. Afterwards, Tom said to me in private that I should be famous and that he could not understand why I was not already well known.

Then he added, "Janet, stay away from Keith. He's heard you play. Believe me, stay away from him. There is *no way* he likes you."

Of course, I did not listen. I attributed Tom's warning to jealousy.

Wanda and I, now both in our mid-twenties, decided it was time to get our own place. I wanted to move downtown. My job was downtown, The Hole was downtown, my *life* was downtown. Accordingly, we moved to a downtown high-rise apartment on August 1, 1989. We moved into Keith's building. Moving there was perhaps the biggest mistake I ever made.

Chapter 21

Within a couple of hours Wanda and I had settled into our new apartment. And what an apartment it was! Beautiful, spacious, luxurious—it was the type of place wherein I had always envisioned myself living. Our ninth-floor, two-bedroom unit with its spectacular view of the city was everything I had dreamed of. I felt that I had arrived, in a way.

We were sharing the apartment with a third girl, Rachel. At the time, the downtown area of Edmonton was the place to be. After scouring this area for weeks, Rachel found us this apartment; and we were lucky to get it. That it was located in Keith's building was the only downside. Whatever. Wanda and I trusted Rachel completely, as Tammy and she were longtime friends and had previously shared an apartment. Granted, our living arrangement was somewhat odd. While Wanda and Rachel claimed the two bedrooms, I lived in the living room. I had a daybed and I used the entrance closet as my personal closet. But I was perfectly happy with this arrangement. I liked the space.

The three of us moved in, unpacked and hit The Hole by 2:00 p.m. Keith and his friends were there when we arrived and were quite surprised to see us. Upon Keith's invitation to join his table, a gesture that was becoming increasingly infrequent, we sat down and ordered a jug of draft beer.

In July, prior to our move, every time I thought of walking away from Keith's circle, either Keith or someone from his group would ask me out to a gig, to a party or to The Watering Hole. And so I moved downtown in the belief that I was a welcome addition to this group. As I was pouring myself a mug of beer, Keith asked me whether I was still planning on attending university in September.

"Yes. Why?" I replied.

"I'm just wondering how you can afford an apartment and school. Wouldn't it have been easier for you to stay home? With your parents?"

I could see where this was heading. Damn! I answered, "Not really. The apartment is closer to the school. And my parents were getting fed up with us [Wanda and me] anyway. We are in our mid-twenties, after all."

"I live with my mother." I had heard that icy tone before, and it still unnerved me.

Silence. Mouth opened, foot inserted.

Finally I said, "But you live with your mother by choice, right? I mean, you could move if you wanted to." And to myself I thought, "Did I get out of that one?"

"Yeah, I guess," Keith conceded, "but how can you afford the apartment and school?" He was not going to let it go.

"I got a big student loan. There's three of us sharing the apartment, so the rent works out cheaper than if Wanda and me shared a two-bedroom, alone." There, that should do it . . . Wrong.

"But why not live on the south side near the school?" he persisted.

Immediately I answered, "I don't know. The south side is not really my thing. It's a little too artsy for me. I like the downtown." Was my mouth still going? "The buildings are newer. Besides, I want to live in a high-rise. The south side is all low buildings. I'm afraid to live in those. They're too easy to rob."

All true. But as much as I tried to explain my having moved into Keith's building, I knew there was nothing I could say that would make it right with him. It was crystal clear that he was not happy with the situation, and I felt foolish, to put it mildly. I felt certain that I had blown it with him big time. My ensuing explanation that it was Rachel, and not I, who had found the apartment sounded lame, even to me. (Rachel left Edmonton at the end of August, leaving Wanda and me in the lurch. I ended up having to pay her share of the rent in addition to mine.)

Deciding it was time to change the subject, I asked, "When is your next gig? Do you know yet?"

"We're playing at the university on Thursday. It's a three-day gig." Yes! The apartment inquisition was over.

"Thursday," I responded. "I guess I'll have to miss that one. I still have to work this month." My job with the provincial government was to end the last week of August. Having attended a Thursday gig once and having suffered at work the following day, I had decided to limit my late night outings to weekends only.

"So come and leave early," he insisted.

Keith wanted me at his gig! Maybe I had not blown it after all. I decided I had better show up that Thursday or risk losing him completely—like I ever had him to begin with—so I agreed to go.

The conversation then shifted away from us, and Wanda and I went home to our new apartment. Once in the apartment, I thought, "Screw it! I like my apartment and I'm staying. Keith will have to learn to live with it, like it or not."

And the bar sang its sweet song of welcome, and I embraced its subtle ambiance . . . and chugged back a cold   one . . . (Yeah, yeah, I'm turning all poetic again.)

Living in the apartment a hop-skip away from The Hole, I soon found myself residing at the bar. My two-drink limit remained in effect, but I felt drawn to the bar almost daily. And I mean *drawn*. My mania compelled me to go there, for I was fulfilling God's plan, The Plan. Also, I discovered early on that living in an apartment is not quite the same as living in a house. For whatever reasons, when you live in an apartment, you want to be away from it as much as possible. At least I did. And with its earthy charm, The Watering Hole was comfortable.

Beer is life; life is beer
Beer is golden—like the sun
　　And wet—like the rain
　　Hence life, hence growth
Beer has a head; people have heads
Beer is life; life is beer.

Poem "Beer" © 1990, J. M. Knudsen

(That one just came out off the top of my head. Not all poetry is serious.)

Now that I was living downtown, Doreen and I began to hang out together on a daily basis. Doreen believed in New Age religions and New Age philosophies. She embraced Buddhism and Wicca equally, and she followed tarot cards. I recall her saying that "when three good people get together, the three form a powerful, holy circle; and the tarot cards then speak the truth." Wanda, Doreen and I formed such a circle, according to Doreen. She further explained that the "power of three" was well known and dated back to the most ancient of cultures.

Wanda only *played* with the tarot cards. She did not believe in them as having power or influence. Certainly, I was skeptical when it came to the tarot—or any form of fortune-telling, for that matter. I was skeptical until our daily readings, which we did in my apartment, began to come true. We would anticipate who would show up where, and what—if anything—might happen . . . and we were *always* right! It never dawned on me that someone might be eavesdropping at my apartment door. In fact, I deemed the notion of eavesdroppers paranoid.

Doreen and I went to The Smoking Guns' Thursday gig as promised. We stayed for the whole show and continued on to The Hole afterward. Despite the knowledge that I would suffer at work the next day, I could not leave. I was having too much fun, and I was too much in love.

At The Hole, Doreen and I got a table together. Keith did not acknowledge us at all. I had already begun to think that he was freezing me out of his life, and this exclusion only served to further my belief.

Grasping at straws, I asked Doreen whether it was normal for Keith and his crowd to exclude *her* from their circle.

"Yes," Doreen replied. "Sometimes the band just wants to be alone to discuss business."

"But Doreen," I returned, "if that's true, why are Leah and Yvette sitting with them?"

"Those two are like sisters to Keith," Doreen replied without hesitation. "He told me that himself."

" 'Sisters' who sleep with him?" I had to ask.

Doreen laughed. "Sleep with Keith? Where did you get that idea? He's never slept with them." Her matter-of-fact tone was reassuring.

"Why do you say that?" I pressed.

"Because he told me," Doreen asserted. "Besides, everyone knows Keith's in love with you."

That was what I wanted to hear. And for one whole second, I was happy. Ecstatic.

Whatever bond I may have formed with Leah, Yvette and the other girls in Keith's entourage had broken by the end of July. My belief was that all of the girls liked Mr. Jones and therefore hated me. All of the men in Keith's circle of friends, however, continued to be friendly towards me. They flirted with me outrageously! And I thoroughly enjoyed their overtures. They boosted my self-esteem to a level wherein I felt both beautiful and desirable. The icing on the cake was that Keith appeared completely angry, jealous, whenever his friends flirted with me. His jealousy was the confirmation I sought, the proof that he did love me.

I went to the Friday gig at the university with Wanda and my old friend Trish. I remember asking Trish, whom I deemed an impartial observer, whether it was true that Keith did indeed stare at me all the time while I danced.

After watching him all that night, Trish declared, "You're right about that. He *does* stare at you a lot."

That was what I needed to hear. I now believed it possible that Keith did have feelings for me. Actually, my brain was like a seesaw when it came to Mr. Jones: up, he loves me; down, he loves me not. The ensuing cycle of ecstasy and despair fed my illness. I was steadily falling deeper and deeper into mania, going to a place that I had not yet been—the realm of delusions and voices. But it took awhile to get to that frightening, lonely place.

In August 1989 The Guns' crowd continued to get together for Saturday afternoon baseball games. At one such game I met Lars. He was the sole member of this crowd whom I had heard of but had not yet met. The reason we had not met became apparent to me soon enough. While we were playing, out of nowhere Lars shouted at the top of his lungs, "Satan is lord!"

I was utterly horrified! Was he joking? If so, I did not get the joke. The rest of the players looked equally surprised. I had heard correctly and I did not like what I had heard. Not at all.

Later, in 1990, I realized that Lars was the boy from The Asylum who had relentlessly taunted me over Sherry's death. The three SOBs were now together again, all grown up: Hank and Jerry from the Hell House parties, and now Lars.

Lars' one statement at the baseball game had a tremendous impact on me in the long run. Ultimately, I wondered whether everyone I had met in Keith's crowd worshipped Satan.

Doreen was sick. She became sick first. At one of the baseball games she said to me, "Janet, it never rains on you."

I looked at her quizzically.

Pointing up at the sky, she repeated, "It never rains on you."

Instantly the clouds, which had been heavy and gray, parted; and sunshine poured over us.

With my eyes on the sky, I responded, "It's probably just a coincidence, Doreen. Anyway, I've gotten soaked in the rain many times in my life."

But Doreen insisted, saying, "Since I've known you, it hasn't rained on *you*. Keith has noticed it too."

"What do you mean?" I was trying hard to make some sense of what she was saying.

"Keith told me it used to rain on his gigs all the time and that since you've come around, it doesn't [rain]."

I still would not lend credence to what Doreen had said. It

was too crazy, too weird. Of course it rained on me. It rains on everyone.

Another day, Doreen asked me if I noticed "the numbers."

Clueless as to what she was talking about, I asked, "What numbers?"

She then explained that for each day there was a specific number that symbolized that day's vibration. The number gave you a general insight into what kind of day that it would be: good, bad, mediocre. The more you understood the numbers, the greater your insight would be. She now asked me to try to feel the number.

Thinking, "Sure, why not?" I looked around my apartment where my gaze repeatedly landed upon 2s. I saw the number 2 on my digital clock, I saw the 2 on my television, and I was drawn to items placed in pairs on my shelves. Finally, I looked at Doreen and said, "Two. I think the number is two."

Doreen was overjoyed! She said that I was correct and that I was the first person she had ever met who could see the number. From this day forward, whenever Doreen would ask me what the number was, I always responded correctly.

Doreen was very sick. But I did not recognize her illness. I knew nothing about mental illness.

Next, Doreen asked me if I noticed "the colors."

Mulling over her question, I replied, "Everywhere I go, I see black and royal blue. They're my two favorite colors, which is probably why I've noticed them."

Again Doreen was ecstatic. She, too, had seen the colors. She was truly happy to discover that she was not alone in her thinking.

Doreen made a final revelation: "Janet, it's all one."

I was absolutely baffled—not that it was "all one," but that someone other than me had seen the oneness.

She explained, "It's all one and it all relates to you and Keith. Everything relates to you and Keith being together."

I had no response to that. I was still sane enough to find Doreen somewhat eccentric. She decided she would explain the oneness as it occurred. She was totally convinced that the world revolved around Keith and me. I knew that I saw a oneness; having an ally only served to strengthen my belief in it.

And the oneness of it all began to entrench itself into my thoughts, my brain, my every waking moment. My mania grew.

Chapter 22

That Keith and his group welcomed me one day and shunned me the next became a trend in August 1989. The "friend/not friend" part of The Game was being played out fully. Knowing of my strong faith in God and Jesus, Keith's crowd sported crosses all of the time thus making me believe that they, too, were spiritual. Copying me by wearing crosses was the mirroring part of The Game enacted . . . and it was very cruel. To play upon the thing I held most dear, my love of God, was low. To gain my trust by using God was unconscionable. I would have walked away from this crowd early on if I had thought they were not godly. I am certain I would have left if I had thought them Satanists. But I did not see through it—I saw only the crosses.

If I had even the slightest inkling that Keith's crowd was playing mind games, I attributed the thought to paranoia. I kept telling myself, "That's paranoid, you're being paranoid. There is no game." In my desire for this crowd to like me, I was trapped. But I prayed to God every night to help me. I never stopped praying to Him.

One afternoon in August Doreen and I went to The Watering Hole, and to my surprise Keith came into the bar, *alone*. I had not seen him *sans* entourage in ages. Upon Doreen's invitation to join us, Keith pulled up a chair and we talked.

"So Janet," he said, "I hear The Stones are playing in BC

[British Columbia] in a couple of months."

"Yes, I know. I'm planning on going." Of course I was going. We were talking about The Rolling Stones, after all!

"But isn't that expensive?"

"Yeah, it's around four hundred dollars, but it's worth it," I said adamantly. "I have to see The Stones before they quit!"

"But it isn't wise to spend that kind of money on one gig. What if you need it for school?" Where was Keith going with this? What was it to him if I went to see The Stones?

"I'm not too worried about it, Keith," I replied. "I never worry about money. God always takes care of me money-wise." And that was true.

"Still, Janet," he persisted, "I think you should reconsider. Four hundred dollars is a lot of money."

"Maybe so," I countered, "but the odds of The Stones playing Edmonton are extremely low. I mean, I wouldn't come here if I was famous." (Edmonton is a three-hour drive north of Calgary, Alberta, where the larger and more famous bands usually played. Also, at that time I was not particularly happy living in Edmonton. However, my view of the city, which was then tainted by my depression, has since changed. I now find Edmonton a beautiful city and am very happy living here . . . I am home.)

"Thanks a lot. I guess I'm wasting my time, then." Shit! I pissed him off *again*!

"No, Keith." I had to think fast to salvage this mess. "You tour. That's smart. And you have to live somewhere. Edmonton *is* cheaper than most cities. But . . . maybe . . . I won't go to The Stones concert. You *are* right. It's a lot of money for one night."

There was a momentary lull in the conversation. Changing the subject, I blurted out, "I love your hat!" Keith was wearing a cool black hat that suited him well, just as Charlie had worn way back when. Only I did not remember Charlie now.

"I picked up this hat in Toronto. You really like it?" He smiled as he talked. Finally, he was smiling.

"Yes," I said matter-of-factly. "It looks good on you. You should wear it on stage."

"I will." With that, he excused himself, saying he had to go meet someone.

Doreen and I later conferred that Keith did not want me to leave him, not even for a weekend. And so I did not go to see The Rolling Stones in BC. No, I went to see The Smoking Guns instead. Clearly, I was sick.

Meow! Hiss . . . the claws have come out.

When we first met, Keith and I talked to each other happily. Granted, most of our talks turned into arguments, but at least we spoke, and I kind of liked the arguing. I enjoyed our differences. Opposites attract, so they say, and to me the arguments represented passion. Over the next couple of months the talking petered out to nothing, and all I was left with was his constant staring at me, and . . . I began to think that he was speaking to me through his songs. Everything he wanted to say to me was said through music. I felt that someone, some ominous force, was preventing him from talking to me directly. I had graduated from ecstasy to paranoia, but it took awhile.

I must mention that Keith's following me everywhere I went— from bar to bar, from club to club, from party to party—contributed greatly to my belief that he was in love with me. Even when I went to see his competition play, he showed up. Many people in his crowd told me that Keith *never* went to see the competition; that is, until I came along.

The Saturday baseball games continued in August. At long last, I talked my sister Wanda into going to a game. Just after we finished playing, when the crowd was more or less grouped together, Wanda announced: "The Berlin Wall is coming down! And it will be very warm this winter as a sign that The Wall is coming down!"

To myself I thought, "What the hell is she doing? They're going to think we're nuts!"

But Wanda's predictions registered with everyone at the game, and her predictions proved to be dead on the money. Throughout the usually cold months of October, November and December, it was warm—above freezing—what I like to call, leather jacket weather. And as everyone knows, the Berlin Wall was opened in November 1989 and torn down in 1990. When this prediction was realized,

Keith and his circle began to fear Wanda and me. Up until January 1990, however, Keith's circle held all of the good cards.

At The Watering Hole one evening after Wanda's predictions, Keith invited me to join his table. He did not speak to me except to say "Janet, I hear The Bangles broke up." (The Bangles were a successful, all-girl band.) He then stared at me as if to imply that there was more to his statement, that I understood what he *really* meant by it.

With that one statement I began to believe that Keith was "speaking in code." Clearly, his declaration regarding The Bangles was a direct reference to the fact that our two identical bangles were once again separated, my having returned his bangle—the collateral—to him. Prior to this statement I guessed that he and his crowd were speaking in code. Afterwards I was convinced that a very real code existed. This bangle story is a prime example of the oneness of it all.

Late one night at the end of August, Keith invited me to his apartment. He extended an invitation to Tom, the Confessor, as well. When we arrived at his place, it was just the three of us. I was unaware that Keith's mother was in the apartment in her bedroom. Naturally, I wished that Tom would leave thereby giving me a moment alone with Keith. It seemed that I never got to be alone with Keith anymore, a fact that bothered me enormously. I was always wondering, "Why? Why would they [Keith's entourage] not leave us alone? Why did they have to ruin everything?"

For once, my wish came true. Tom left. Then Keith sat down on the sofa close beside me and said, "Do you believe in 'Romeo and Juliet'?"

At first I did not understand.

"Do you believe in true love?" His eyes locked onto mine. His voice was tender. I could not recall the last time his voice had been tender, gentle.

"Yes, of course," I responded, wondering what he would say next. Was that the sound of my heart beating? It was so loud!

"Do you believe some people want to ruin it for people who have found true love? That's what I meant about 'Romeo and Juliet.'"

I never had the chance to answer. Keith's mother came into

the living room at this moment and ordered me to leave. She did not care for me and had already made that obvious to me on prior occasions. I left, and the tears flowed like never before. But I thought, "Keith loves me! That was his way of telling me that he *does* love me."

The Game: Keith's songs were about me. The Game: I believed he loved me. The Game: I believed we were "Romeo and Juliet." The Game: I was sure that some ominous force was keeping us apart. *It was all The Game.*

At The Hole in early October, Keith played a solo gig and sang to me the entire evening. His eyes never once left mine. That night he sang a song that I dubbed "the proposal song." This was my favorite song. This was the Bob Dylan song I had heard at The Asylum all those years ago: *You Ain't Goin' Nowhere.* Because the song mentions a bride and because I was already ill, I thought that Keith was proposing to me through this song.

By this time I was very sick. So sick, in fact, that I walked away from my university one day and never went back. Now, my parents began to believe that something was wrong with me, but they did not know anything about mental illness. All they knew was that for me to leave university, after trying so long and so hard to get back into school, was not normal. Although they phoned me often, I kept our conversations short. I thought that they, too, were trying to break up Keith and me. I thought the *whole world* was trying to keep us apart. Yes, I was sick.

Despite my mania, despite my illness, I managed to retain some grasp on reality. I was always telling Doreen that maybe we were wrong and that maybe Keith hated me and wanted me gone. Indeed, one day in my apartment I said to Doreen, "If Keith loved me, he'd do something tangible. He would ask me out on a date. That's normal!"

And with this logic I might have escaped the quagmire. I might have walked away, sanity intact. But it was not meant to be. I spoke to Keith that same day and he said, "Janet, if I love a girl, I do something *tangible*. I ask her out on a date." These were his exact words.

After conferring with Doreen, she and I came to the conclusion that Keith was speaking in code once again. His having reiterated my words so precisely meant that he loved me.

Logic had always been my forté. Twisted logic was a skill I mastered after being around Keith for months on end. I needed my twisted logic in order to explain his strange, "loves-me, loves-me-not" behavior. I needed to believe in the code. The code meant that he was in love with me, and I wanted so badly for that to be true.

The Game fed my belief that Keith loved me. The tarot card readings performed by Wanda, Doreen and I always came true. I felt that God Himself was speaking to me through the cards.

Consistent with The Game, Keith and his crowd perpetually repeated words or statements that I had made in the privacy of my apartment. I thought these repetitions were clear indications that Keith still loved me and that I should trust in his love and be patient. I never seriously considered the notion that people could be eavesdropping or that a mind game existed. Even when I did catch members of Keith's crowd listening outside my apartment door, I used my twisted logic to condone their actions. I decided that they were eavesdropping for the greater good, with noble intent.

The most important element of The Game: Keith did everything I asked. Have you seen or read *The Princess Bride*? In it the heroine asks her suitor to do this and that, and the suitor always responds, "As you wish." No matter what is asked of him, he responds, "As you wish," and then fulfills the request. Keith, like the suitor in this story, did all that I asked.

One day I said, "If Keith loves me, he will wear his black hat as a sign."

He wore the black hat faithfully.

Another day I said, "If Keith loves me, he will cut his hair short."

Although he had long, dark hair that suited him well, he cut his hair short.

Next I said, "If Keith really loves me, he will leave Yvette."

Keith had been dating Yvette for about a month. He broke up with her that same day.

And on it goes, my wish was his command except for one

very important consideration: Keith would not talk to me. He sang to me, but he would not *talk* to me.

Where was my head? By the end of October 1989 I thought that Keith and I were embroiled in some big Plan that was connected to God Himself. I thought that we were a modern-day Mary and Joseph and that the evil people in the world would do anything and everything to keep us apart. I believed some of Keith's entourage were the "chosen ones" and that it was their job to keep the evil at bay. The chosen ones, by definition, were those who wanted Keith and me to be together so that God's Plan would be fulfilled. Ultimately, what I deemed God's Plan turned out to be The Game—their Game.

Doreen, who was close to me throughout these months in which The Game was played out fully, became very sick by November. In her psychotic state, she was more observant than the norm. For example, she had already remarked to me that at whatever bar or club we visited, a penny was ever present on the floor at our table, and she was right. Also, she had noticed that there was a preponderance of single-ring phone calls to my apartment. She interpreted these calls to be signals that we *must* go to The Hole, to a gig or to whatever place was on the agenda that day involving Keith and his circle.

One day out of the blue, Doreen and I were nursing drinks at The Watering Hole, and she would not talk to me. At all. She put a finger over her mouth, pointed at the mirrored walls and mouthed, "Sh! The walls have ears."

"The walls have ears"? Instantly I thought, "She's paranoid." After considering her statement carefully, though, I found myself wondering whether people were eavesdropping on me—not just at my apartment, but at The Hole, too. This notion scared me. It scared me because it made sense. It was true that Keith and his crowd repeated statements I had made only at The Hole. "How is that possible?" I wondered. "How big is this game? How many people are trying to keep Keith and me apart?"

On our way out, Doreen pointed at the phones located at the entrance to the bar and whispered, "The phones are tapped."

Again I mulled over her words. It was true that every time I went to The Hole—or any public place, for that matter—there was always someone on the phone. Even Wanda had remarked on the number of phone calls made when we were present at any restaurant, bar or gig. Furthermore, I had to concede that Keith and company repeated statements that I had made on the telephone only. The final nail in the coffin: within a couple of weeks of Doreen's assertion regarding the phones at The Hole, the telephone lines at The Watering Hole and for the next few blocks near it were "repaired." I saw the telephone company trucks. I saw the workers.

When Wanda and I publicly stated that we believed the phones at The Hole to be tapped, Keith and his friends ceased to use the phones in question. In addition, they all spoke more and more softly, if at all, while at The Hole. And they looked *afraid*. If phone taps were a part of The Game, Keith and his pals did not initiate them. Someone else was listening in on us. Someone with money, connections and power.

At the end of November 1989 Doreen was taken to the psych ward and was diagnosed schizophrenic. I never saw her again.

Wanda, at this time, had become paranoid. She did not trust anyone outside of our family.

Another young man we knew from Keith's circle was diagnosed manic depressive.

And me? By the end of November I fully believed in the phone taps and the eavesdropping, only on a much larger scale. My contention was that the media were following Keith and me. It seemed that anything I mentioned in my apartment, on the telephone or in a public place became news within a day or two of my having mentioned it. If I said, for example, "I'm breaking out in hives" (I'm choosing an off-the-wall topic on purpose), the news media would do segments on hives: what causes them and how to get rid of them. Was I psychic? Psychic to the extreme? Perhaps. I do not know. What I am sure of is that I saw numbers, connections and oneness constantly. My mind could not rest.

In a nutshell . . .

"In a nutshell"—is that ever politically incorrect!

. . . Keith and his entourage were following me, and the media were following them, following me. Was I paranoid? Not quite. I was still trying to convince myself that everything was coincidental. But by Christmas the seemingly infinite number of coincidences broke me down. I became paranoid. In my delusional state I believed that every song, every movie, every book and every television show was somehow about Keith and me. I fully believed the world revolved around us . . . around me.

And until March 1990, I continued to believe in Keith's love for me. I did not care who was following us—the world could follow us!—it did not matter. As long as I loved Keith and he loved me, everything would work out fine.

Chapter 23

I played my first paying gig at The Watering Hole at the end of November 1989. It was just me and my guitar—solo, as the cab driver had predicted so many years ago. I remember the painstaking effort I put into arranging my set lists to achieve a necessary oneness. That neither Keith nor anyone from his circle showed up for my gig hurt me tremendously. Although I did not understand their absence, I played well. The show must go on.

Who said that? Why must the show go on? Why not say "Sorry, but I have to disappoint all five of you . . ." OK, my audience numbered around 15, but still I felt alone.

I did have some support in the audience that night. My sister Wanda came to the gig along with Trish, who was accompanied by her new boyfriend, Brendan. Brendan was tall, handsome and nice. I liked him immediately and deemed Trish lucky to have found him. My affinity for him probably stemmed from his being a stranger to me and from the knowledge that he was unacquainted with Keith and company. Also, Brendan played bass guitar. A musician, like me.

After the show, which did go over well, I went home to my apartment and pondered why no one from Keith's crowd had shown up. And then, using my twisted logic, I reasoned that Keith could not support my career. To do so would be proof that he did love me, and our love had to remain a secret for the moment. It would be dangerous for Keith if the men and women in high places guessed or knew that he did love me. The secret had to remain intact to ensure that God's Plan would be realized.

In December 1989 The Game changed dramatically. Throughout the Christmas season Wanda and I were invited to several house parties and gigs. The same people who had been ignoring us since the end of October extended these invitations. Keith's crowd had become very friendly again with one glaring exception: Keith would not talk to me.

One house party in particular stands out in my mind. At this party I sat on a couch with Wanda. When Keith arrived, he sat directly across from me and stared at me all night. He did not talk to me. He did not talk to anyone, really. The tension between us was palpable— so much so that everyone at this party talked quietly, if at all. I recall the looks he and I received. People looked back and forth, from Keith to me, as if to say "Talk! Say something! Anything!" I would not break the silence. Pride would not allow me to speak first. And Keith had become a master at the art of remaining silent. We had once again reached our now usual impasse. Yet I felt strangely calm. I kept thinking to myself, "God's Plan is working. Don't worry, be happy."

Upon returning to our apartment, Wanda asked me whether I had noticed the large, upside-down black cross in one of the rooms at the house party. I told her that I vaguely remembered seeing it and asked why it concerned her. She replied, "That cross is satanic. Don't you know anything? They're Satanists, Janet!"

"No, Wanda. You're wrong!" I was certain that she was wrong. After all, Keith and his friends all wore crosses, and Keith mentioned God in his songs. No, Wanda had to be wrong.

Being deeply manic, I felt that this Christmas was especially holy because God and His chosen ones were together at last. His Plan was being fulfilled right in front of me. I was at long last becoming a professional musician. I was deeply in love with the man of my dreams. I could hear God daily through the numbers and through the constant barrage of messages and codes I found everywhere I looked. I could not turn my head without seeing some symbol, some sign, some message from God telling me that I was on the right path, His path. Finally, I was certain that Keith would come to me on New Year's Eve and that our union would signal a new beginning for the world. As one, we would usher in a time of peace.

New Year's Eve came and went. The Smoking Guns played a gig that night in which they were the opening act. That Wanda and I were in attendance goes without saying. I took great care to achieve the right look for this momentous occasion. I wore a black Lycra mini-dress with a sheer lavender scarf around my shoulders. I sprinkled silver glitter in my hair and on my body. Ethereal. I wanted to look ethereal. I suppose I did.

I remember feeling sad that night. Even before I left my apartment, some part of me knew that Keith would not come to me. Oh, but I hoped and prayed I was wrong. He had to love me. Right? My love could not have been in vain. Not again. This thing between Keith and me—it was God's Plan. It was all about us, just like Neil Young sang:

> *Well, I dreamed I saw the silver*
> *Space ships flying*
> *In the yellow haze of the sun,*
> *There were children crying*
> *And colors flying*
> *All around the chosen ones.*
> *All in a dream, all in a dream*
> *The loading had begun.*
> *They were flying Mother Nature's*
> *Silver seed to a new home in the sun.*

> *Excerpt from song "After the Gold Rush"*
> *© 1970, Neil Young*
> *Cotillion Music Inc. & Broken Arrow Music Corp.*

When the clock struck twelve, I left the gig. Actually, I walked away from the party while the clock was still chiming in the hour. I managed to hold back my tears until I reached my car. It would not do to have anyone see me crying. A porcelain doll does not cry. It breaks, but it does not cry.

Up until this night I felt certain that there was a plan from God involving Keith and me and that this plan was working. My faith in God—and in Keith—was unshakable. Praying fervently later that night, I asked God, "What's going on? Please tell me so that I can understand. I *don't* understand."

For the next few days, I operated in a fog of confusion and despair. I considered suicide time and time again. I hated the way I was feeling. Continuous, sustained hopelessness was new to me, and I could not stand it. My mania was such that I could not accept the reality of my life, the reality that Keith did not love me. Instead, I decided that maybe I had made a mistake: I was correct in thinking Keith loved me but wrong about the date when we would be reunited for all eternity. My thoughts now turned towards suicide. If Keith did not love me, then I would kill myself. I had suffered enough for one lifetime.

And then I had a truly psychic moment. On January 5, 1990, I thought, "Call your old boss. They will give you back your job." The job to which I am referring is the clerical position I had had with the provincial government. This was the job I had left at the end of August to pursue my university education.

With supreme confidence I phoned my old supervisor. She said, "Actually, it's funny you called me today because someone just quit, and I was just about to post the position." She then told me that I could start back immediately. Because of this psychic moment my faith in God and The Plan was fully restored. God had talked to me and I had heard Him correctly. That was that.

Going back to work was good for me. At work, I could not spend every waking hour looking for signs and obsessing about Keith. I did, however, see the numbers like never before. Over time, the numbers took on meanings.

A "2" signified that I, accompanied by one other person, would have a nice time were I to go out. A "3" meant that I would go out with two other people and have a marvelous time. A "5" indicated that I *must* go to The Hole. Lastly, a "6" was a sign that were I to go out on the town, it would be an expensive and miserable outing.

In the beginning, I saw only those four numbers: 2, 3, 5 and 6. As time went by I added both "11," which stood for extreme anger, and "7," which represented the destruction of evil, to the list. The last number I saw was "32." I have no idea what it means, but I still see 32s everywhere, every day, even now. My best guess is that 32 represents this book.

I describe the numbers because when I met other manic-depressives, I learned that they, too, saw numbers and equated meanings to the numbers. Interestingly, although our interpretations of the numbers might differ, we were in agreement regarding whether a number was positive or negative.

After New Year's Eve turned out to be a bust, I set a new D-Day, or Decision-Day, in my mind. Keith would have to profess his love for me by Friday, March 23, 1990, or I would be forced to concede that he was playing some sort of vicious mind game on me.

My gig at The Watering Hole was the first of many solo gigs I played. In the ensuing months, I pursued my musical career wholeheartedly, phoning every lounge in the city and finding at least two weekend gigs per month. I earned as much as $100.00 per night for my playing. Only once did a member of Keith's crowd attend a gig. As for Mr. Jones, he never did show up.

As D-Day neared, I became increasingly manic depressed. Being both sky high and suicidal on the same day was not unusual. At home and at The Hole, I began uttering threats of suicide. I said, "If Keith doesn't love me by D-Day, I'll kill myself. I'll jump off the balcony." Although I cried often, I always wore a smile in public. At The Hole, I threatened suicide with an unshakable, unbreakable smile on my face.

I took great care not to mention the actual D-Day, March 23, out loud. After all, if Keith loved me and was truly one with me, he would know the date psychically. By this time the media were "following" me to the point that I was becoming afraid to say anything out loud. No matter what I discussed with Wanda in the privacy of our apartment, it became news within a day or two. The media would pick up on a word or a phrase or a topic and repeat it to an extreme that it became noticeable. Wanda, too, noticed these repetitions. Ultimately, she and I resorted to writing each other notes to communicate any ideas that we wished to have remain private. We both believed that our apartment was bugged and that our telephone was tapped. How else could the media know everything we discussed? Wanda also noticed the single-ring phone calls to our apartment that occurred almost daily. We changed our phone number two times, getting unlisted phone numbers both times, to no avail.

By this time Wanda believed that most of Keith's crowd were Satanists. She was convinced the single-ring phone calls, the pennies on the floors at bars and the repeated code words or phrases were all satanic spells to get us to go out. At first, I did not agree with her. At first, I thought Wanda was paranoid.

The pot calling the kettle black, or what!

Did you know that one major difference between mania and schizophrenia is that those diagnosed with the former illness can understand and interpret phrases like "the pot calling the kettle black"? A schizophrenic would tend to take the phrase literally; that is, a schizophrenic would think the pot was actually talking to the kettle. Interesting.

On Friday, March 23, 1990, I got up and went to work as usual. All day long I prayed that Keith would come to me that evening. All day long I worried that what was my God's Plan was in reality their Satan's Game. And all day long I wondered what I would do if I were wrong and had been wrong all along. Keith had up until 7:00 p.m. to come to me, "7" representing the destruction of evil and therefore at one with God's Plan.

When I arrived home from work, I remained in my apartment. Over and over I cried, "I'm going to kill myself. If Keith doesn't talk to me today, I'm going to kill myself. He *has* to love me. Doesn't he?"

Seven o'clock came and went. Finally, having to face reality, I broke down. The sadness I felt, however, was quickly surpassed by anger—anger that I had been used, anger that so many people had played this horrible mind game on me. But my anger was nonviolent. Many people equate mental illness with violence, and they are so wrong. This stigma exists because all we ever hear about in the media are those cases involving sociopaths or violent psychotics. A quiet, pacifistic mentally ill person is not newsworthy, after all. The truth is that studies have revealed that patients who were pacifists before mental illness set in remain pacifists afterwards. For the most part, even when I was delusional, I did not become violent (although I instinctively felt the need to protect myself during the Big Breakdown of 1993). There was *never* any compulsion for me to kill someone. Just the opposite. Believing that everyone wanted me dead, I became completely terrified of people. My instinct, therefore, was not to hurt anyone but rather to hide away from the world.

Thanks to my anger, I did not kill myself.
Well, there's a statement of the obvious!

Instead, Wanda and I went to see The Alley Boys' gig at the university that same night. Sure enough, Keith and his entourage were there when we arrived. He and his friends could not hide their shock or fear upon seeing me. And I knew then that they had believed me when I said that I would kill myself. Even though I had been voicing suicidal notions since New Year's Eve, not one person in Keith's entourage had stepped forward to tell me the truth. Not one had said, "Janet, Keith's playing with your head. We're playing a game." Not one had admitted to having known me in Montreal. I was shattered.

> *What fun! You've come undone*
> *In pieces on the floor*
> *But in time, you finally find*
> *There's so much less to more*
> *Yeah, there's really nothing like before.*

Excerpt from song "What Fun!" ©1991, J. M. Knudsen

I had to show him . . . I had to show all of them that they meant *nothing* to me, so I danced the night away with a smile pasted on my face. The porcelain doll had returned.

Later that night I concluded that there was a mind game, The Game. The conversation about suicide that I had had with Keith months earlier was his way of feeling me out—he was trying to determine whether I would kill myself. And so I finally discovered The Game's objective: to destroy my faith in God and thereby lead me to suicide.

I was horrified, sad, alone and lost. But God had made me a fighter.

Chapter 24

That I was not the only victim of The Game became apparent over time. I later learned that there had been several suicides and mental breakdowns among the alternative crowd and that live mind games were a constant with this group. These games follow a basic pattern in which the players enact a part, or role, and perform specified actions in order to score "points." The actions are aimed at a designated "target" who is then barraged by constant head games initiated by the players. What I call The Game is actually a combination of several different types of mind games. I believe The Game is worldwide and its players all know each other in the sense that they are members of a deadly club.

The first and most crucial part of the mind game is to befriend the target. Once trust is established, the target becomes easy prey. The cruelty of The Game is readily apparent. Targets crack up— become manic, depressed, schizophrenic—or commit suicide, never realizing they have been used. They never know that their so-called friends have played a deadly game on them.

We hear about suicide among teenagers all the time. As the years go by, the age of suicide victims is becoming younger, leaving family and friends of the victims with one question: Why?

I believe no one decides that life is not worth living without help, without being given a push. This push comes from the cliques that abound at school, at work and in social settings. If you are not part of the clique, you are deemed against it; and you therefore become a potential target. I have already discussed the components of The Game, but they bear repetition: the "I don't know you" game, repetitious questions, mimicry, mirroring, following or stalking, eavesdropping, the "friend/not friend" ploy and the fact that The Game never ends. Once a target, always a target.

Does all this sound paranoid? Of course it does, and therein lies the dilemma faced by targets. If you believe yourself a target, you appear paranoid. And if you say "I think someone is out to get me," you will most certainly be labeled "paranoid." The victims of The Game are stuck between a rock and a hard place. I have described The Game so that its victims will know that they are not alone and that it is *not* just their imagination.

Even the strongest person can break under the pressure of these mind games, especially when that pressure is constant, never ending. Targets, more often than not, are the strong people. They are the people who do just fine on their own. They are the people who do not need a clique to tell them how wonderful and hip and cool they are. And the cliques know exactly how to destroy them.

The Game initiated by the cliques has been refined over time into a type of science. The only real defense against The Game is the realization that it exists and that you may be a target. If you think you are a target, examine your friends closely. Are they hot and cold towards you? Do they want to know all about you, while they reveal very little about themselves? Do they show up everywhere you go? Are they friendly with you in private, while they ignore you in public settings? Consider these questions carefully. If you answer them honestly, you will know whether or not your friends are true friends.

One more note about The Game: I believe The Game drives some youngsters towards violent behavior; hence the current onslaught of school killing sprees.

So March 23, 1990, I awoke to the realization that everything I had thought in relation to Keith and me was a game, a vicious game. And in my naiveté I still did not and could not believe that anyone could be that cruel. In my mind, I therefore attempted to justify both Keith's actions and the actions of his entourage. For a moment, I entertained the notion that some other member of Keith's group loved me and that Keith was acting as a shield for this other man, but the futility of this line of reasoning was readily apparent to me. To myself I thought, "If a man loved me, he would tell me. That's reality."

Given this thought, I was forced to admit to myself that everything to do with Keith and me had been a mind game in which I had been an all too willing, gullible target. The rape had left me in a position of needing to be loved. As such, from the beginning I was more than willing to believe Keith loved me, and over time my sanity demanded that he did. The cruelty of his actions, his pretending to love me, was unthinkable to me and was the proverbial straw that broke the camel's back.

About a week after D-Day, Wanda and I returned to The Watering Hole. Naturally—or should I say, unnaturally—I wore my mask. Tom, the Confessor, joined us immediately. The first thing he said was, "I knew you guys would win."

Puzzled, I looked at him and asked, "Win? What did we win?"

"The Game," he replied. "You guys won The Game."

Rather than ask what game he was talking about, I decided to play along that I knew the game to which he had referred, hoping he would give me more information about it.

"It was really close at the end," Tom continued, "but Lars and I knew you'd win. We were the only two who bet on you."

"Bet"? The word rang loudly in my mind. Bet?! People, some with whom I was not even acquainted, had been betting on me? The rage I felt at this moment was greater than any anger I had ever felt over anything in my life. Remaining outwardly calm, I said icily, "Of course I won. I'm smarter than all of them put together."

"You're not all that smart," Tom needled. "After all, it took you this long to figure out they were faking it."

Still oh so calm I retorted, "How do you know? Perhaps *I've* been faking it from the start. Have you ever considered the possibility that I was playing a game on them?" With that remark, I turned the tables on them. Now they would always have to wonder whether *they* had been used.

"No way . . . I don't think so . . ." Tom's voice was no longer confident, cocky.

"Believe what you want," I continued. "All I know is that they look like scum to everyone who saw them and their game, and I look like an innocent victim. When people realize that Keith did not love me, they're going to be mad!"

After all these months of Keith's following me and staring at me all lovey-dovey, most of the people on the scene believed Keith loved me. In fact, many strangers on the scene had approached me asking *me* why I was being so mean to *him*. I remember one girl, a stranger, asking, "Why won't you talk to him? He loves you. It's obvious. Just look at his face when he sings to you."

My response to her and to anyone else who questioned me about Keith was, "No, he hates me." And I said this believing that part of God's Plan required that the love Keith and I shared had to remain secret until the right time arrived.

Talking to Tom, I continued, "Keith just destroyed his own career in music. No one is going to want to go near a guy who plays mean head games. And I promise you, everyone on the scene will know there was a game!" With that, the conversation ended.

Over the next couple of months I talked about The Game everywhere I went, taking care not to name names. Although I discussed The Game with Wanda only, I spoke just loud enough so that anyone who wanted to listen, could. Naturally, I no longer went to Keith's gigs whether he was playing solo or with his band. And I soon learned that slowly but surely his audience was dwindling.

Still angry, I began to believe that there had been more people at Keith's gigs to watch me dance than had been there to hear his music. OK, that sounds egotistical and may not be right, but I have been told more than once that I am a pretty good dancer, and . . . I had noticed that a lot of men stared at me when I danced at The Guns' gigs.

For a good year, everywhere I went on the scene, people asked me, "Are you going to The Guns' next gig?"

My reply: "No, I don't go near them anymore." I did not

elaborate why.

Keeping abreast of what was going on with Keith and his career in the following year, I discovered that he was having difficulties maintaining a steady lineup of players in his band and that his venues were growing smaller and smaller.

*Hah! What goes around **does** come around. Vindictive? Bitter? Hell, yes! At first, anyway.*

From D-Day until mid-May I continued to work for the provincial government. And I worked hard to appear normal, sane. I was fully aware that much of my thinking at this time was paranoid, so I did my best to ensure that no one knew about my paranoia—the paranoia that was becoming increasingly real as time went on.

You get the picture. I was paranoid that people would think I was paranoid because of my paranoia. (I just laughed at this one.)

I was terrified that "they" would lock me up and throw away the key.

At work, my coworkers remarked that I seemed unusually chipper, when all the while I was killing myself just trying to keep it together. My hope was that by looking and acting happy, I would feel happy. Unaware that I was losing my mind, I could not stop my descent into insanity, nor could I figure out a way to hold onto my happiness. My mind would not, could not, rest.

An interesting point about mental illness: you do not know you are losing your mind—your sanity!—for the first time, until you have already lost it. That is, even though I knew I had paranoid thoughts, I still deemed myself sane even *after* I believed in my paranoia. Only when I went to the psych ward and was administered antipsychotic drugs did I realize that I had been completely out of it, insane. In my case, however, now that I am familiar with the symptoms and signs of my mania, I know my best course of action is to contact my psychiatrist immediately whenever these signs appear. With his help I have been able to curb my mania, which always begins with ecstasy and extreme energy, before it grows into the dreaded paranoia, delusions and voices that ensue when I am not properly medicated.

With the closing of my department in May 1990, my job ended. Although I was offered a position in another department, I did not last very long. My illness had finally succeeded in making it impossible for me to work; a forty-hour workweek was no longer viable. I lacked the strength and focus necessary to hold onto a normal job. My thoughts were occupied with a million different ideas, none of which related to work—or to life in the real world, for that matter.

Because of my loss of income Wanda and I were forced to move to a one-bedroom apartment. After an extensive search for an apartment in the downtown zone, we chose to remain in our current building, Keith's building.

In the next few months I turned my attention towards music and my solo career, hoping that I could make a living playing lounges. And I began to write songs. In summer I tried my hand at "busking," playing my guitar and singing on street corners with my guitar case open to collect tips. Keeping busy at all times was a must. I had to occupy my mind fully in order to escape the despair and paranoia that threatened to take over my life.

Throughout the months following D-Day, a smile was engraved on my face. To remind Keith and his pals that their game had failed, I continued to frequent The Hole. Indeed, my pride dictated that I go to The Hole and act happy while there so that Keith would never know how much he had hurt me. So I resided at The Hole. And I was consumed with one thought, one question: "Why?" Why had Keith played a game on me? What had I done to deserve such heinous treatment? I needed to know why! The idea that he and his friends had been cruel to me for the sole purpose of being cruel was preposterous to me.

Although I appeared happy in public, I was crying all the time in private. For whatever reasons, in July 1990 I began to think about the rape. Specifically, I pondered the visit I had made to the clinic in August 1988 a week after the rape. My mind then seized upon the notion that I had been given an abortion without my consent. In reality a D & C was performed, but at this time all I could remember about the clinic was that a local anesthetic had been administered so that the doctor could do something. Now growing increasingly paranoid, I firmly believed that the "something" was an abortion. I decided to determine whether I was correct. I had to see my medical file.

Accordingly, Wanda and I went to the clinic in question, and I asked the nurse at the reception desk if I could see my file. She pulled my file and told me the date of my last visit. When I asked to look at the file to read it for myself and see the charges that had been billed to it, the nurse refused. She said, "We do not give out files. Under the law, you are not entitled to that information. All I can tell you is when you were last here and which doctor you saw."

I argued with her. "But what did he [the doctor] do that day? He did some kind of surgery. I know he gave me a local."

Finally the nurse responded, "He performed a D & C with your permission. I have a signed consent form."

Still anxious to read the file myself, I said, "Fine. Just let me see what the file says."

Again, she refused.

Not knowing what a D & C was, I left the clinic absolutely convinced that I had been given an abortion without my consent. Convinced. The nurse's treatment of me at this clinic pushed me over the edge. My paranoia now became my reality.

I grieved over the perceived abortion throughout the summer months. The sadness that stemmed from it pierced my soul and left a gaping wound that stitches could not heal. The idea that I had undergone an abortion caused me far more pain that the rape ever could. I could no longer stop my tears. My sadness was there for everyone to see. At long last, the mask was gone.

In September, now fully paranoid, I put garbage bags over all the windows in the apartment that Wanda and I shared. I was afraid people were spying on me. Between The Game, the rape and the perceived abortion, I fell off the tightrope. However, I still knew my paranoid thoughts had to remain my secret. That fear of being locked up was always in the forefront of my mind when dealing with people. Only Wanda knew what I was really thinking. As she was sick, too, she could not help me.

Despite my illness, I went out and played gigs and busked regularly that September. There was one highlight that actually gave me a moment of joy. One Saturday afternoon I was playing a gig at a country and western lounge. A gentleman visiting from Oklahoma gave me a twenty-dollar tip and said, "Darlin, your talent is wasted here. You belong in Nashville." This was the greatest encouragement I had ever received in relation to my music from someone outside of my family.

I agreed with this gentleman in one respect: it was time to move!

I wanted out of Edmonton badly. To that end, Wanda and I sold all of our furniture with the intention of moving to Vancouver, British Columbia. I kept only my guitars, my jewelry, my clothes and my car. Not surprisingly, at the last minute I changed my mind about moving. Instead, I gathered up all the cash I had made from my part of the sale, and I bought myself an expensive six-string guitar—a Guild guitar whose sound quality is unsurpassed in my estimation. At night I now slept on the living room floor, but I did not give a damn! I had a great guitar! Finally, I had the kind of guitar I had dreamed of, and playing my Guild gave me some much needed joy.

After Wanda and I sold off everything we owned, my parents realized we were not well. But not knowing anything about mental illness, they did not realize how sick we were. They did not put it together that we could be mentally ill. Wanda's illness was mild in comparison to mine, but she was paranoid nonetheless. As for me, my mom has told me repeatedly that she simply could not believe I could be sick. After all, I was the one with the genius IQ. I was the one who was good at everything and who would therefore achieve great success in life. How could I be mentally ill?

Thinking that a break from everyone and everything might do the trick, my parents gave Wanda and me enough money to go on a weekend vacation away from Edmonton. We drove to Drumheller, Alberta, and spent three wonderful, peaceful days there. Drumheller is the home of a large dinosaur museum and is renowned for both this museum and its badlands. While in Drumheller I wrote a song called *Still*:

Tired eyes, see the loveless gather 'round
Looking for some safe new ground on which to rest their
                    gaze . . .
Tired of lies, hoping that a love can last in a world that spins
                    too fast
To start again.

                    Excerpt from song "Still" © 1990, J. M. Knudsen

When Wanda and I returned to Edmonton, our parents bought us some new furniture. And Wanda and I decided we had to move out of our building, Keith's building. For my part, I needed to feel safe. I needed to know that nobody could eavesdrop or spy on me. The constant paranoia had to stop!

Chapter 25

On October 1, 1990, Wanda and I moved to another downtown high-rise apartment. The rent was a little cheaper and was more in line with our combined incomes. Once again we rented a one-bedroom unit, and I continued to live in the living room. The two-bedroom units were out of our price range. The building itself had beautiful hardwood floors and an old-fashioned charm that appealed to me. Most importantly, I was more comfortable here than I had been in our previous building. I no longer had to worry about Keith and his crowd having access to my apartment.

Because Wanda and I remained paranoid, my parents bought us some black-out curtains that eliminated our fear that people were looking into our apartment. And thanks to the new furniture my parents had bought us, this apartment felt like home in no time. I could relax— a little, anyway.

At this time I was living on unemployment insurance and was trying to earn money playing occasional gigs. But by the end of October, I was so weakened by the sadness I felt over The Game that I could hardly muster up the energy required to lift up my guitar. Depression does that to your body; it physically depletes you of your energy and strength.

Because of the lingering sadness I felt over the rape and the perceived abortion, I phoned the police that same month to discuss the rape. The officer I spoke to was extremely nice and compassionate. He asked me to come into the police station as soon as possible so that he could question me further about the rape.

I went to the station the following day. The officer asked me to describe in general what had occurred the night of the rape. I explained the event as best I could, telling him that I had said "No" to Jack many times over, that night. The officer then emphasized that "No" meant "No!" And based on my having said "No," he concluded that I was an unwilling participant and that, indeed, I had been raped. He further added that the fact that I had been cut on the hymen and had bled for several hours was sufficient information to indicate that it had been rape. He then asked me why I had waited so long to report the rape.

I responded that at that time I did not know for sure whether what had happened constituted a rape. Furthermore, I really did not want anyone to know what had transpired because I was embarrassed, ashamed. I certainly did not want my parents to know about the rape, because I thought they would be hurt badly, and I did not want to cause them any pain.

The officer then asked me why I felt that it might not have been rape.

I replied, "I was dizzy that night. I had had three drinks and I could hardly walk. I thought maybe I did something to lead Jack on."

The officer responded once again that "No means no" whether drunk, stoned or sober. He indicated that it sounded to him like I had been drugged that night, and he then added that the rapist was liable to repeat his crime.

"Because the rape occurred more than two years ago," the officer stated, "you would not win in court if we charged this guy. However, if you write a report describing the details of the incident, we will keep the report on file. That way, if the SOB tries to do it again, the case against him will be strong."

Then he looked at me, his compassion evident, and asked, "Can you do this? Can you write a statement for us?"

I told him I would. As soon as I got home I wrote my report, which I submitted to the police the next day. In taking this action against the rapist, I felt much better. Now I was armed with the knowledge that I had done something to try to stop Jack from repeating his crime. Writing and submitting this report gave me back some strength—it empowered me. I regret that I did not take action against Jack at the time of the rape. Perhaps I would not have gotten as sick as I did. Who knows?

Once in our new apartment, Wanda and I determined to stay away from The Watering Hole, from Keith and from his friends. I was still wondering why Keith and his pals had played their game. I simply could not let it go. Finding a reason for their cruelty was essential. I kept asking God, "Why?"

One day out of the blue, I picked up a pen and paper and let my mind wander on the page. I wanted to see what I would write were I to clear my mind of all thoughts and just write whatever came out. This "automatic writing" is known to psychiatrists and psychologists and is sometimes used as a tool to delve deeper into a person's psyche.

I drew a baseball diamond and a kite. Instantly, the name Sherry came into my mind. Seizing upon this name, I recalled in full the baseball murder from so long ago. At last, some of the puzzle pieces were falling into place. Keith and his crowd were the kids from The Asylum. In the very least, they were connected to the kids from The Asylum. Some of them had been at the deadly baseball game. One of them had bludgeoned Sherry with a bat.

And so I understood The Game: Keith and company wanted me dead or insane because they thought I had witnessed Sherry's murder.

It is clear that I may be wrong about my conclusion, that Sherry's murder may be something my brain concocted. But my conclusion did answer my "why" at the time.

Once I realized that Keith and his group were all from Montreal—or had lived there at some point in their lives—everything made sense to me. All signs pointed to one major conclusion: Keith and his friends were Satanists. Wanda had been correct all along. They were Satanists. They believed in spells and ritual sacrifices and lethal head games. They were *true* Satanists.

In all my life I had never believed in the existence of Satanism. I guess I had lived a sheltered life. In my naiveté, I had never given any credence to the existence of Satanists, witches or evil cults. Because I could not accept that anyone could be so foolish as to worship the Devil, I did not believe in satanic cults. Therefore, the realization that Satanism was a reality proved traumatic for me.

The recollection of Sherry's murder prompted me to reflect on Montreal and my childhood there. I had true memories of seeing a burning cross at a park and of listening to news reports about missing, murdered or raped children. In my now paranoid state, however, I began to experience what I call "false memories"—delusional recollections that felt like very real remembrances. I now believed I had seen numerous satanic ritual killings, Sherry's murder among them.

My paranoia was as logical as it was crazy. My logical explanations of perceived traumatic events only served to heighten my paranoia and make my paranoid thoughts more and more real to me. I had many vivid false memories that seemed quite real, true, at this time.

I thought that when I was 3 years old, I had seen a satanic ritual at a nearby church in which cloaked figures drank blood from a severed baby's head. I further believed that when I was 5, I had seen cloaked figures sever the fingers of two young children, Anna and David, and place the fingers in a jar of beets. The fingers were to be used to create a "hand of glory," which is a satanic thing about which I know nothing other than its name.

Of note, in my mind virtually all of the victims of the satanic rituals that I believed I had witnessed had names (like Sherry, Anna and David), which furthered my thinking that these ritual sacrifices had, in fact, occurred and were all too real.

At the time of Sherry's death, two other young girls were reported missing. I now firmly believed that the three girls' disappearances were related. My logic suggested that these girls had seen some sort of satanic ritual and were therefore murdered.

Finally, I thought that Keith had an older sister who, too, had been murdered or sacrificed. Her name was Laurie, and the saga created in my mind about Laurie is worth telling. Again, I emphasize that this was a false memory. And still, to this day, the memory feels very real. But I do now know that it was a paranoid delusion, as were all of the murders I have just described . . . with the exception of Sherry's murder. For reasons I know not, I still believe Sherry was murdered in the way I have described. I am actually afraid to look into the matter.

I met Laurie in the summer of 1976 at the pinball arcade I frequented at the time. I was approaching my 12th birthday. With her miniskirts, cowboy boots and short hair, Laurie stood out in the crowd. Her western attire was definitely unique for Montreal. I remember thinking that I wanted to look like her when I was older, and ultimately I did. Laurie told me that she was from the West Island area of the city. She came to my neighborhood to see her boyfriend and was often accompanied by her brother, Keith. Keith told me that Laurie was special, that she was the chosen one. When I asked him to elaborate on what he meant by "chosen one," he said, "She will be Satan's bride."

I could not believe my ears. Had I heard him correctly? Again I asked Keith to elaborate. He explained that Satan had chosen Laurie to be his bride and that the wedding was to take place in a few days. He added that Satanists throughout the world were excited because they thought the wedding would bring Satan to Earth where he could rule over and reward his followers.

I asked, "How does this wedding work, exactly?"

Keith replied that Laurie would be sacrificed to Satan in a wedding ritual, and then both she and Satan would rise from Hell and commence their rule on Earth.

I said nothing. I wanted to talk to Laurie directly to see if she knew what her wedding entailed. And as soon as Keith left, I did talk to her.

Laurie informed me that she did know about the ritual death and that she was looking forward to her special day. She explained that she had been chosen from a group of eligible 12-year-old girls through the sacred match game. In this game the match lady, a chief witch, had held matchsticks in her hand and had let the girls select one match each. Having chosen the longest match, Laurie had won the "honor" of becoming Satan's bride.

I tried my best to convince Laurie that she was wrong, that

she would die and not come back. But she did not believe me. A week later, Laurie was murdered.

So, this story about Laurie sounds and is insane. But I deemed it real at the time, as did I the other sacrifices I have described. I was so positive these events had occurred that I wrote up reports on these murders and submitted my reports to the police. Fortunately, the police then contacted my parents and explained to them that they thought I was mentally ill and in need of psychiatric help.

But I was not ready to be helped. I was in a quandary as to whether my parents were good or evil.

Basically, I believed that my parents knew who Keith was—that Keith was someone I had known in Montreal—and that they had not told me. I felt betrayed, at first. But then I reasoned that my parents *could not* tell me about Keith, because they knew the Satanists had placed bugs in their house and taps on their phones. Furthermore, because of a story my dad had told me about his mom *playing* with a Ouija board, I thought my grandmother had been a witch when she was alive. I therefore decided that my dad was a good man who had chosen not to follow his satanic family. Of course, this thinking was way out there—I had already kissed the real world goodbye—but my crazy logic insisted that I connect the dots even if I had to make them connect. In other words, if reality did not fit into my puzzle, I twisted it sufficiently that it would fit.

And still I believed the world revolved around me. Just me. No Keith. I decided that the only reason Keith had been followed at all was that he was following *me*, he was hanging around *me*. Key words and phrases I used only in my apartment (no longer in Keith's building) continued to show up on the news. For example, if I said, "It's time to reflect on things," the news would report that "reflection" was required in relation to some news item. I would hear the word "reflect" everywhere. Television shows, songs, news items, magazines, radio—all mentioned the word "reflect." Each time I heard my key word, I was all the more convinced that I was being followed . . . and that God's Plan was working. No longer knowing what God's Plan was did not bother me. I was happy just knowing that His Plan was working.

Ultimately, I decided that I was on this Earth on behalf of God, and Keith on behalf of Satan. The Game was him against me, but The Plan was me against him.

My paranoia grew to the point that I was certain everyone I had met in Alberta was either from Montreal or had lived there at some time. In addition, I believed that I had met every world-famous musician while I lived in Montreal and that I had written the songs for which they were famous. I further thought that I had met every well-known actor, writer, artist and politician while living in Montreal. Montreal was the key, the common thread, the glue that held together all of my delusions.

Delusions of grandeur continue . . .

I believed that I had written a myriad of television shows, movies and books and that I had painted many beautiful works of art. I had accomplished all of these things while still a young child, before my 5th birthday. Essentially, I believed that as a child I had possessed some kind of super brain that enabled me to write an album's worth of music in a day or a year's worth of a television series in a week.

It was all about me . . . everything good in this world had come from me, from my mind. And I knew that everything that came to my mind came from God. In other words, all the creative tasks I believed I had achieved as a child were God's achievements with me acting as His instrument.

So, to me it *was* "all one," and the oneness existed because it had all come from God through me. Logical? Insane?

"All the world's a stage." Because I deemed this Shakespearean line a fact while I was delusional, I could not get this line out of my mind. I felt that the whole world was in on The Game and had chosen sides; some chose Keith and Satan, others chose God and me. In my mind, unseen powers were manipulating events to ensure that my words would be repeated in the media and that my manner of dress would become the "in" fashion. Whereas in the past (back when I was sane) I had attributed everything to coincidence, I now believed I was being followed to show the Satanists that the majority of people in this world supported me and God's Plan. I was being copied so that the Satanists in this world could see that God was the true power. In following me, people were showing that they followed God.

One chilly December evening, my dad showed up at my apartment and invited both Wanda and me out to dinner. After dinner my dad took me to see a psychologist—yes, my parents tricked me into getting help. I discussed both Sherry's murder and The Game with the psychologist. Speaking to my dad in private, the psychologist recommended I see a psychiatrist immediately because he felt certain that I suffered from a chemical imbalance and therefore required psychiatric drugs. (Psychologists are not medical doctors and therefore cannot prescribe drugs.)

Within days of this visit to the psychologist I went to see a psychiatrist. It is incredibly difficult to get an appointment with a psychiatrist. The wait can be as long as six months. I was fortunate in that my psychologist, who felt my situation was urgent, knew a psychiatrist who could be persuaded to see me right away.

I met with the psychiatrist and he prescribed Haldol. Haldol seems to be the medication of choice for the treatment of psychiatric disorders when there is uncertainty as to what the diagnosis is. In my experience, Haldol was the initial prescription I received from three different psychiatrists.

And I took the Haldol . . . at first. But in my deluded state, I eventually believed the drug was a placebo and I therefore disposed of it. My parents knew I had stopped taking my meds—I am not sure how they knew, but they knew—so they came over to my apartment with a replacement prescription. They begged me to take my medication without fail. Because I could see the concern on their faces, I consented to do as they asked. I swallowed my pills. If not for my parents help, I would never have been treated, I would never have recovered. For a long time my parents paid for my meds. Even after I returned to work, I could not afford the drugs that I required to remain sane.

A lot of people are curious as to why mentally ill patients discontinue their medications. There are a number of reasons with which I have had personal experience. First and most importantly, I did not accept that I was sick. Next, I did not believe the meds were working; as I noted, at one point I thought my meds were placebos. Another reason was that while deeply paranoid, I thought the meds were a slow-acting poison designed to kill me gradually so that it would not appear that I had been poisoned. The main reason, in my case, was that I thought the drugs were designed to make me forget the truths I had discovered regarding Satanism—that "they" wanted to control my mind so that I would not remember my past brushes with Satanism and "them." Other reasons included the belief that I was cured and the desire to feel that manic high once more. Those of us suffering from mental illness tend to forget just how bad it was to be sick, paranoid, delusional. The highs, however, remain quite clear in our memories.

At the end of January 1991 Wanda and I moved back to our parents' house. Since both Wanda and I were paranoid, my parents felt they needed to have us in a place where they could closely monitor us.

Because I had paranoia that I had met my psychiatrist in Montreal (and also because I simply did not click with him), I found a new psychiatrist who immediately prescribed Haldol and Cogentin. Taking these drugs, I became semi-sane, at best. Actually, I still had all of my delusions of grandeur. The meds only succeeded in making me sane enough to keep my delusions to myself.

So ends the saga of my first nervous breakdown.

Chapter 26

Moving home was good for me in that I felt safe again. Being manic at the time, I wrote 32 songs in the space of two months. My parents, who enjoyed my original music, decided that I should pursue my musical career and asked me what I required to move ahead. I told them I would need a professional demo tape to submit to the record companies. So, with my dad's backing, I made a tape of four of my favorite songs complete with a hired band of backup musicians. Ultimately, I was disappointed with this tape because the man who mixed the tape failed to bring out my guitar playing. This demo tape, therefore, failed to showcase my talents properly. And I was far too sick to voice my input. Indeed, I was sufficiently paranoid that I ended up believing the man who recorded and mixed my music was out to ruin my career.

I did not and could not work at this time. Between mania, depression and paranoia, I simply could not function properly in society. I was aware that I had suffered a breakdown, of sorts. I define a breakdown as having occurred if I have succumbed to my paranoid delusions to the extreme that I can no longer function in the real world. And in 1991, I was fighting my paranoia. I was trying to discern whether some of my delusions were based in fact, while others truly were delusions. I was in the real world only in that I was aware that some of my thoughts *might* be paranoid.

I sent off my demo tape to a few record companies, but the response was unfavorable. In most cases, the tape was never even heard and was returned to me still sealed in its original envelope. To succeed in the music industry these days, you have to make your own CD, produce a good quality video and tour the country all at your own expense. (This is my understanding of the way things work in the music industry. Of course, there are always exceptions to the rule.) Since I was too sick to follow this route, I gave up on the idea of being a professional musician. Disillusioned as I was, I became severely depressed.

I slept away most of 1991. By April of that year I had no choice but to apply for medical welfare, which meant that the burden of paying for my meds was now removed from my parents; the government would have to look after me. Although I visited my psychiatrist every two to three weeks, I did not feel he was helping me. I faithfully took the Haldol and Cogentin he prescribed, but still I remained ill. All of the paranoid delusions I had endured before seeking psychiatric help remained intact, except now I was questioning their veracity. As time went by, for every delusion I dispelled, I suffered a new delusion to take its place.

These new delusions, false memories, were similar to the previous ones. Basically, I was consumed with the notion that the majority of people in this world were satanic and that I had been the victim of their evils. Despite the meds and my semi-awareness that I could be delusional, my delusions were becoming increasingly horrific, radical, strange, impossible. And of course, I kept all of my delusions, new and old, to myself. My paranoia had grown to the extreme that I trusted only my family, and I could not discuss my delusions even with them.

In the summer of 1991 I suffered from an assortment of horrific, paranoid false memories. I believed that I had been both assaulted and sexually abused as a young child—not by my parents—but by some satanic cult.

In one nightmarish vision I saw myself at age 3 lying on a kitchen table surrounded by cloaked adults, one of whom cut off my genitalia. Among these cloaked adults was a "twin" of my mom. Thankfully, the twin differed from my mom in that the twin had black hair and an expressionless, blank face. In this vision my dad then burst into the room and shot everyone there, including my mom's twin, thus saving me. Somehow, miraculously, a doctor restored my body.

This vision, nightmare, was to me the most upsetting of all the psychotic thoughts with which I now lived. I love my parents more than anyone in this world; in my heart they are second only to God. Therefore, the visions I had involving my parents' "evil twins" were especially terrifying and eventually led to my *worst* breakdown—the Big Breakdown, as I call it.

As a side note, it is only in recent years that I have read and heard about the mutilation of female genitalia. My vision preceded my knowledge of this current-day atrocity.

In another vision—I should just stick to word "nightmare"—I was lying on a table in a small, dark room. I was 3 or 4 years old. The cloaked figures were there again. This time they cut out my tongue, burned out my eyes and cut off my hands and feet. No one came to save me. I prayed to God to restore me and He did. I then left the room under His protection.

Did I believe these nightmares to be real? Yes and no. Even though they felt real, my meds were working sufficiently well that some part of me realized the impossibility of these events having taken place. I was definitely walking on the tightrope once more. Fortunately, my meds kept me from falling off, from losing my sanity completely.

The next nightmare I lived with was also particularly hard on me. In this one I was 9 years old, and I had gone to a friend's house. There I found three adults sitting in the den, preparing to pluck out my friend's eyes as some sort of a satanic offering. I begged them to stop, to which one of the adults replied, "If you will sell your soul to Satan, we will let him [my friend] go."

Since I could not stand to see my friend suffer, I consented to do as asked. I signed over my soul in blood, my blood.

The man who demanded my soul was the evil twin of my father. But for the blank look in his eyes and a lighter hair color, he looked like my dad.

After I had signed the contract, the three adults insisted that I prove my loyalty to Satan. They ordered me to praise Satan out loud and to utter disparaging remarks about God and Jesus. In particular, they wanted me to say "God damn . . ." I did as they demanded because I wanted to live and to escape them. When they finally let me go, I went home and cried and prayed to God to forgive me. The friend later asked me whether I was a Satanist to which I replied, "No!"

The friend said, "But you sold your soul to Satan, you know."

My retort: "Yes, but God bought it back!"

I have described these three nightmarish visions, false memories, in the hopes that people will better understand delusional thinking. I have seen the terror in the eyes of psychotic patients on the psych ward. During one of my stays on the ward, I vividly recall one frightened woman yelling out, "Stay away from me! You're Satan!" to her parents. So I have to believe that many psychotic patients suffer from these same kinds of delusions—delusions that can render you paralyzed with fear, delusions that place you in hell on earth, afraid of *everyone*. It is just you against the satanic world, and the fear that stems from this type of thinking is unimaginable. Short of living it, you cannot possibly comprehend this terror. I fully understand why some psych patients become catatonic. And sadly, I understand why some patients feel the need to protect themselves through violent behavior: extreme fear. Perhaps the most important step in understanding and treating mental illness is the recognition that the patient has these unfounded fears, but fears that are nonetheless very real to the patient.

My other delusions at this time, delusions that do not fall into the category of false memories, were not quite so terrifying. Because I believed Satanists were trying to kill children as part of their sacrifices, I examined my neighborhood public parks. When I noticed that all of the parks I visited had hills, I thought to myself, "If a child were standing on the other side of a hill, I wouldn't be able to see him. He could be abducted, and nobody would see it."

Next, I believed that money from the sale of illicit drugs was the Satanists' chief source of income. To this end, I thought there were underground tunnels throughout the city designed to sneak the illegal drugs into the city. I began to think that architecture was a satanic field.

And was I ever paranoid of people in the medical profession. I was certain that Satanists chose this field in order to have control over those of us who were on God's side. I believed that every baby was born with a twin and that the evil doctors and nurses separated the good twins from their evil counterparts at birth. Being in a hospital, these evil doctors could easily find victims to sacrifice in their satanic rituals. The evil psychiatrists could then ensure that anyone who threatened to expose the Satanists and their atrocities would be locked up. Now do you understand the fear that takes hold of those suffering from paranoia and delusions? Originally, I was not going to include my thoughts on the medical profession; however, these are the very thoughts that led to my worst fears.

Still pondering Keith and the why of The Game, I briefly embraced the notion that Keith was a good man and that someone close to me was evil. I wanted so badly to think that he was good and that he really did love me. Turning my attention towards Wanda, I thought, "What if she's Satan? What if she's the reason Keith couldn't be with me . . . and if she's Satan, then . . . I must be . . . God."

*Now **that** is a delusion of grandeur!*

Fortunately, the love I have for my sister put an end to that line of thinking. In fact, by summer's end I was becoming normal again. I was dispelling many of my bad thoughts and nightmares, and was finally conceding to myself that I might be both paranoid and delusional. I guess it took several months for my meds to kick in, but thankfully by September I was returning to the real world again.

When I began to accept that many of my bad thoughts were imagined, I cried rivers of tears. I wondered how I could be so evil as to think my sister or any member of my family would hurt me. And how could my mind have invented all of those horrific nightmares? How could I have been so evil as to invent those visions? I cried and cried, until one day I saw a sign from God indicating that He had forgiven me. Slowly, I forgave myself and allowed myself to feel happy again. Very slowly.

By December 1991, I was back to being manic. Only this time it was the good mania, the creative mania—tremendous energy and creativity and joie de vivre. I became utterly obsessed with my hair. Bleaching my blue-black hair platinum blonde for a Rod Stewart concert was a must. I also got two new piercings in my ears.

I dyed and dyed until I fried
Hair today, gone tomorrow

After the concert I wanted my hair to be black again. It did not work out that way. Instead, I killed my hair and was left with no choice but to cut it all off like a crew cut. Oh well. There are worse things.

And in December, a new thought came into my life. Pondering reincarnation, I decided that I was the reincarnation of Marilyn Monroe. I had never given credence to the possibility of returning to this world after death. But now I was certain that reincarnation was real and that I had been Marilyn in my former life. My guess is that I picked her because she looked like she had had a sad life, especially when it came to love. I could definitely relate to that.

I loved the Rod Stewart concert, by the way. It was great!

Chapter 27

The year 1992 was a good one for me. It was a year of relative sanity, and it afforded me the opportunity to rebuild my strength.

Despite the effectiveness of my meds I continued to cling to some of my paranoid notions, and I continued to keep this paranoia to myself. My psychiatrist was ever in the dark when it came to what I was really thinking. I still felt that the world was somehow eavesdropping on me, perhaps through bugs and phone taps. My fashions continued to set the trend. Whatever style I adopted was soon emulated throughout the world. I was absolutely convinced that the police were following me everywhere I went to protect me from the Satanists. And the numbers continued to be a part of my everyday life. Indeed, I was still somewhat ruled by the numbers and their meanings.

On the plus side, the nightmarish visions were no longer in the forefront of my thoughts. Although I was not yet totally convinced that all of my false memories were fictional, I did choose *not* to think about them anymore. I decided to tell myself that the murders, mutilations and abuses I had envisioned were all nightmares and were best forgotten.

When my psychiatrist felt that I was well enough to work again, he prescribed a course of action to enable me to find work.

Because I had been unemployed for so long, from May 1990 to April 1992, my psychiatrist recommended that I contact a local organization whose sole purpose was to help employ those who had been off the job market for long periods as a result of mental or physical illness. I went to the required meetings with this organization and found a full-time job the following week. Naturally, I did not tell the company that hired me the nature of my illness. I felt certain that I would not have been hired if the company knew from the start that my illness was mental and not physical.

I believe there is more stigma attached to mental illness than to any other illness or disease. And why is that? My contention is that people fear the unknown, that there is insufficient information available to the public regarding what mental illness is. I know that before I fell sick, when I heard the word "psychotic," I immediately thought, "violent." And I am sure that most people today are guilty of this same incorrect association. Guess what I have discovered since having fallen ill? Every time I disclose to someone that I have manic depression, I learn that the person with whom I am speaking either suffers from mental illness personally or has a friend or relative who suffers from mental illness. The illness is widespread. The illness is silent. It is time to talk!

I was hired as a data entry clerk at a low starting salary. Knowing that my odds of finding a better job were nil, I accepted the position. I went from earning $12.00 per hour with my government job to $8.00 per hour in this private industry position. Having no job benefits, I had to pay for my meds out of my own pocket. Luckily, at this time I was more sane than not, but my lack of medical benefits later proved detrimental to my recovery. My salary dictated that I take the lower priced meds available; my illness, however, dictated that I take the newer and more costly meds on the market. My sanity was directly dependent upon my income.

The company that hired me was connected to the housing industry. As such, my job was particularly laborious in the warmer months. Within a few days I mastered my data entry job of typing up work orders. About a month into the job, another girl quit and I was promoted to her position of quotations clerk. Given the difficulties involved in my new position, I succeeded in talking my boss into a dollar-per-hour pay raise. I now split my days between preparing quotations and typing up work orders. My one friend at work was an older lady who, like me, did data entry and who, like me, smoked.

I was happy enough with my job. Within two weeks of being hired, I went out and bought myself a brand new car. My old car was finished, dead, so I required a new vehicle to get me to and from my workplace. Buying a new car both cheered me up and gave me the incentive to hold onto my job. More importantly, buying a car helped me to feel like a regular, functioning member of society.

By November 1992 work had slowed down tremendously. Because there were no quotes and no work orders, I was perpetually being sent home after putting in a half-day's work. There was simply nothing for me to do. Needless to say, I was not happy with this situation. I had been hired with the understanding that my position was to be full time, eight hours a day, year round. Even without the car payments to which I was obligated, I could not afford to live on half of my full-time income. Were I not living with my parents at this time, I do not know how I would have survived. My parents allowed me to live rent-free pending the restoration of my full-time salary. Without my family, I would have ended up homeless.

As Christmas was approaching, my job died out altogether. Accordingly, the company gave me a temporary layoff with the promise that I would be recalled once business improved. Once again I was forced to go back on unemployment insurance.

When Wanda and I moved back to our parents' house at the end of January 1991, we stopped going out; that is, we avoided the nightclub and bar scenes completely. I spent my evenings knitting or doing needlepoint. And I simply did not give a damn if I ever went out again. Keith and his game had effectively taken away all the fun of going out. Unwilling to run the risk of bumping into any of The Game's players, who continually frequented the night scene, I chose to stay home. To distance myself even further from Keith and memories related to him, I cut my hair very short and dyed it red. Now when I saw my reflection, I was not the Janet who loved Keith. Instead, I was a new me . . . and a sad me.

Then I noticed an ad in the entertainment news for a band whose name rang a bell. The ad stated that this band would be playing at The Diner, my old haunt, on a Tuesday in December. Assuming the band's lineup had not changed, the bass player, Brendan, was the ex-boyfriend of my old friend Trish. (She had left Edmonton back in 1990.) Since I had always liked Brendan, I decided to take a chance and go to see the band. Wanda agreed to go with me as she, too, liked Brendan and his crowd.

When Wanda and I arrived at The Diner, we were happy to find Brendan on the stage playing his bass. He smiled at us immediately, making us feel both welcome and happy. On his break he came over to our table to chat. I soon learned that he was still single and not currently seeing anyone, so I took a chance. A big chance. I gave him my telephone number, leaving it up to him to call me. He did. The very next evening he called and invited me out to a movie. We went to see Bram Stoker's *Dracula*, a movie I love even now.

At the end of our date, Brendan invited me to a house party for the coming Saturday night. I went to this party and enjoyed myself. Meeting new people felt good. I had been antisocial for so long that I had forgotten how much I enjoyed meeting, learning about and getting to know new people. My relationship with Brendan progressed rapidly—too rapidly, as it turned out.

Because I was still on my layoff and because Brendan worked approximately five hours a day, he and I saw a lot of each other in the ensuing months. I spent many days and nights at his country home located 45 minutes away from the city by car. And . . . I let him convince me to stop taking my antipsychotics. I also stopped seeing my psychiatrist. The fact is that I felt normal, sane. Maybe my previous mental problems were just a one-time-only thing. It was possible . . .

Brendan was a health nut. He firmly believed that all I needed to do to be well was to eat proper meals and drink fortified fruit and vegetable juices. He meant well—and I was well, for a while. I was changing, too.

For the first time since I was 20 years old, I let my hair go back to its natural brown color, and I decided to let it grow long.

Brendan was very much into the natural look. I was inclined to please him. Besides, I hated the red hair! My makeup changed as well. I now wore only eyeliner and lipstick, a look that remains with me even today.

In the middle of February 1993, I was called back to work. Knowing I would be seeing less of Brendan, I was at first saddened by my job recall. But at the same time, I knew that I had to get on with my life and return to the real world. That same month, Wanda and I moved to an apartment near our parents' house. Once again we were sharing a large one-bedroom unit with me living in the living room. Having my own place again helped me to feel more normal. After all, most 28-year-olds did not live with mom and dad.

Once I had moved into my own place and returned to work, Brendan's interest in me slowly died away. My worst fear was being realized: I was going to be alone again. I hated to think it, but I soon conceded to myself that Brendan had been more interested in my car than in me. While I was unemployed and virtually living at his place, I had let him have carte blanche with my vehicle. Now that my car and I were no longer at his beck and call, he did not want me. I took it hard.

Instead of accepting that the relationship was over, I became needy and obsessive over Brendan. And sad. In trying to hold onto Brendan, I was really trying to hold onto my sanity. I knew I did not love him, but I also knew that I did not want to lose him. I saw him maybe twice a month after I moved to my own place. The writing was on the wall; I chose to look at the floor.

At work, things were good for about one month. The older lady whom I liked failed to show up at the office one day. One day became a week, a week became a month . . . she never came back. And the company failed to replace her. It was spring, the busy season, and I was now doing both her job and mine. Granted, I was good at my job—I was always fast and accurate—but the stress of typing up all of the incoming work orders while continuing to prepare quotations eventually proved too much for me and for my sanity.

While employed with this company, I spent my lunch breaks alone in my car. In those half-hour breaks, I smoked three cigarettes and pondered God, The Game and Brendan. I did automatic writing constantly, obsessively. The writing would indicate that "All is well" and that "God's Plan is working." The writing kept me going. The burdens of my failing relationship and my stressful job were eased somewhat by the belief that God's Plan was, indeed, working.

In June 1993 I decided to take charge of my relationship with Brendan. First, I dyed my hair blue black and cut it short. No longer was I going to try to be Brendan's ideal woman. Back in black, I was Janet the rebel once again. To me, the black hair was and is symbolic that I am fine on my own and that I am strong.

Next, I met with Brendan and said, "I think we should just be friends." I said it first! God knows I had heard that phrase enough times in my life. Brendan quickly agreed. He was overjoyed that I had reached this decision to be friends. I was, of course, heartbroken, but at least now I knew where I stood. Or did I? The very next time I saw Brendan he made sexual advances towards me, and I therefore assumed that our relationship was on again. By July, however, I was forced to accept that he and I were finished. Our relationship over, I became severely depressed.

What I refer to as the Big Breakdown began that July. I had been off of my meds since having met Brendan in December 1992, and for six months I had functioned as a relatively sane, normal person. No one knew I was sick, least of all, me. No sooner did I lose Brendan than my thoughts returned to Keith . . . again.

By now you must think me pathetic. However, I absolutely believed that Keith was my one and only soulmate. Even while things were good with Brendan, my thoughts often strayed towards Mr. Jones. I still felt that things were unfinished between Keith and me.

Why, oh why can't I find closure? I need closure, man! (Valley girl accent.)

I now thought that maybe I had been mistaken about Keith and The Game. Once again I believed Keith did love me and that our time had not yet arrived. In thinking Keith was good, I had to conclude that other people were evil. These evil people in the world knew that Keith and I belonged together and would do anything and everything to keep us apart.

I had a vision wherein I was in Hell, and I shouted out "God!" at the top of my lungs. Immediately, Keith came into Hell and put his black coat around me, shielding me completely so that I could no longer see the evil and suffering of Hell. He then plucked me out of Hell and brought me to Heaven. Keith was God. I had been Satan. In imagining every terror and horror possible, I—once God—had placed myself in Hell. Whereas Keith, as God, had remained pure in thought and deed, I had strayed into the realm of evil in my imagination. Evil therefore became a reality. In short, it was my fault that evil existed. But Keith, God, forgave me. And realizing that forgiveness is essential to love, I forgave myself. In my uniting with Keith, we were God, mother and father, once again. Such was my vision and my reality.

I believed everyone in the world knew that Keith and I were God. Some people, the chosen ones, were with us; most were against us. The media were following us, so much so that I felt I could not breathe without the world knowing that I had taken a breath. "All the world's a stage" echoed in my mind continually as a reminder that the world was the playground in which God and Satan's war was being waged. I believed everyone on Earth had chosen to come to Earth to play The Game. Keith and I had created Earth for the sole purpose of providing a neutral place in which to carry out our—God's—Plan. All of the souls on Earth had come from either Heaven or Hell. Whereas the souls from Heaven had volunteered to come to Earth, the souls from Hell had no choice but to come. The Game *was* God's Plan! They were one!

When Keith, God, had saved me from Hell, a new Satan whom I named "Max" took over the rule of Hell. Max was truly evil. My evil had existed in thought only; Max's evils were enacted. When God forgave me my sins, He forgave the world. I was the first soul to be forgiven. And as God, I believed in love and forgiveness, and I preached repentance. Having suffered the terrors of Hell, I wanted to save the world, to save every soul. I therefore devised a plan with Keith, God's Plan—The Plan. We would create a place wherein all souls, good or bad, would live together. Keith would play the part of Satan, having chosen to do so. I would be God. Together we would work to bring Max's followers back to God. Our main objective was to save Max's soul and thereby save Max's followers; thus all souls would be saved and would be returned to Heaven for all eternity.

Our plan necessitated that the media follow us. Everyone had to know what Keith and I were doing, and we each had to know what the other was doing. The good souls working in the media would ensure that I, God, was followed and that Keith, Satan, was ignored or ridiculed. In other words, the media would work to show everyone that following God resulted in happiness, while Satan's path led to misery.

There was one key aspect of The Plan that all souls would know. Keith would come to this Earth knowing who he was—God in the role of Satan—and knowing his purpose. I, as God, would not know anything about The Plan. I was going to prove that faith in and love for God were all that one needed to be happy. Through the power of God's love, I would win The Game and fulfill The Plan.

And so this is the scenario I created in my manic mind.

It almost sounds real, doesn't it . . . almost?

Chapter 28

I do not know why, but at this time—and in all my manic phases afterwards—I found myself repeating four famous quotations to myself over and over and over: "All the world's a stage," "Vanity, thy name is woman," "Hell hath no fury like a woman scorned," and "That which does not destroy me makes me stronger." Having pondered these quotations now that I am healthy, I believe I have some idea as to their significance.

"All the world's a stage" related to The Game. "Vanity, thy name is woman" was related to my obsession with my outward appearance, an obsession that stemmed directly from my not feeling inwardly beautiful. All of my dark thoughts weighed upon my conscience, and I blamed myself for having imagined the terrors I have described. "Hell hath no fury like a woman scorned" is a phrase that strengthened me in my weakest moments. Anger makes me fight, and fighting to remain sane is the most difficult fight I have ever encountered. I thank God that I have been victorious in this battle. And the line that helped me to keep on keeping on was "That which does not destroy me makes me stronger." I have to think I have surpassed even Hercules in strength by now.

In the second week of July 1993 I started hearing voices. My auditory hallucinations started innocently enough. One day, while sitting in my car during my lunch break, I thought, "If God is talking to me through signs and symbols and codes, why can't He just talk to me directly?"

Immediately a female voice said, "Hello Janet."

Mentally, I replied, "Hello. Who are you?"

I never spoke out loud when conversing with my voices. I was aware that I had to appear normal at all costs. Fitting in, in the real world was ever present in my thoughts; that is, I knew my thoughts and actions could be labeled "psychotic."

The voice answered, "Carol. I'm your guide. I'm glad you finally asked to talk to me. I've been waiting for you. I've been with you all along."

Carol and I talked continually from that moment on, up until I decided she was evil.

In reference to The Game and God's Plan, one thing in particular plagued me: why had I forgotten everyone? Despite my many encounters with Keith and his crowd over the years, I did not recognize or remember any of them from one meeting to the next. Why?!

I did not feel that the trauma of Sherry's murder explained my inability to recognize Keith and company. Upon obsessing over this enigma, I reached a conclusion that I deemed viable. I believed that I had been hypnotized to forget anyone and everyone satanic or somehow connected to Satanism. I had forgotten all of my horrific visions because of hypnosis. And the key to my hypnosis was the color blue. As long as I saw blue, I would not remember anyone or anything satanic that I had encountered in my life. I determined that the Satanists chose blue because blue is my favorite color. This perceived hypnosis provided me with an answer that could explain away any glitch I may have had in my manic perceptions of the world, in my version of reality.

Returning momentarily to the oneness of it all, I thought the reason that David Letterman regularly said "*I been hypmotized [sic]*" during his television show was to help *me* remember *my* hypnosis. Yes, Dave was definitely a chosen one. He was on my side.

Keith's role was pivotal in breaking the hypnotic spell that I had been under for so long. Only he could shake me out of my slumber and force me to remember him and The Plan. Essentially, Keith had treated me with extreme cruelty so that I would awaken to the realization that evil does exist. And once my mind accepted that evil is a very real presence in this world, I tore down the walls I had built to shield myself from everyone and everything bad. In my naiveté, I had believed without a shadow of a doubt that "no one could be that cruel" in reference to Keith and his "loves-me, hates-me" mind game. In accepting that Keith *had been* that cruel to me, the hypnotic spell that I was under was broken. I now remembered everything!

I felt certain that many celebrities were on my side—not just Dave. Musicians were writing songs with lyrics designed to help me remember the past. Movies contained lines or plots or even props to jiggle my memory. The world was working diligently to help me remember that Keith and I were God and that we had come to this Earth to play out a game. A game designed to save souls. Knowing that the whole world was helping me to remember the many satanic atrocities I had seen or survived made me feel extremely loved . . . and needed. It was beyond wonderful to believe that so many people loved me and wanted to help me, Janet. I was utterly euphoric!

I could easily forgive everyone any evil that had been done to me. I could not, however, so easily forgive crimes against others. As a strong individual, I felt I could handle any evil including rape, torture and mutilation. In my mind, I had interceded on behalf of innocents on many occasions, making myself the victim of numerous unspeakable horrors in order to save others. My purpose on Earth was twofold: I had to protect the innocent, and I had to find Max. Part of The Game and The Plan was that I identify Max, a puzzle only I could solve.

My euphoric vision of the world and The Game was nice while it lasted. It did not last long . . .

Even in my insanity something always happens to ruin my happiness. Shit!

In the middle of July 1993 I bought eight binders and 1200 sheets of paper, thinking I was supposed to write a book—a really, really big book—about God. My book would prove God exists using nothing but logic and would thereby be my instrument to save the world. I wrote nothing. I was waiting for divine inspiration and trusted that I would write the book at the right time.

The single-ring phone calls that had plagued Wanda and me since 1989 continued on a daily basis. These calls were supposed to keep me hypnotized. Now aware that the calls were one of many satanic spells, I was no longer fazed by them. Indeed, none of the satanic spells—pennies on the floor, code words, single-ring phone calls—worked on me anymore. I was free! Finally, I was awake!

I was so awake that I could not sleep. My mind kept rolling over The Plan. I was perpetually thinking and rethinking everything that had happened and everything that had been said relative to Keith and his circle. Of course, my thoughts at this time were a mishmash of reality and perceived reality. Nonetheless, putting it all together, making it all one, consumed me. I was trying desperately to figure out the identity of Max, the real Satan. I slept no more than three hours a day, on a good day. Automatic writing had become an obsession now. For hours on end, I wrote about the assorted terrors that I believed I had seen or endured. Virtually all of my waking hours were spent writing.

These new terrors, false memories, were truly horrific and made my earlier nightmarish visions seem benign. In one vision in which I was 8 years old, I had been forced to have sex with a boy I knew, while adult spectators filmed this sex act. Other new terrors centered on sodomy and bestiality. But the worst of the new terrors involved evil twins. I had visions in which my sisters' evil twins had tried to murder me. I had a waking nightmare in which the evil twin of my father had abused me while the evil twin of my mother had watched and cheered. The Satanists had used my family's evil twins against me, knowing that they could destroy my sanity in so doing. In short, the Satanists wanted me to become evil and to join them. Their chief objective was to render me, God the mother, evil. And they wanted me in their ranks because they wanted my—God's—power.

But I fought against my nightmares. I clung to reality with all my might, telling myself over and over that "My family loves me," and "My family is good." I reminded myself that were I to give in to the Satanists and allow myself to believe that my family was evil, I would lose The Game. God's Plan would be destroyed.

MY FAMILY NEVER HURT ME! THAT IS REALITY!

Thinking about this part of my breakdown makes me sad. So sad, in fact, that I put off writing this part for days. My family is completely loving and supportive, and they have always been my rock. God and my family are my "reason to be," as I put it. I later told my current psychiatrist that one thought in particular had driven me over the edge, had made me lose my mind: the belief that my family was evil.

By the last week of July, I lost my sanity. I had built a large house of cards in my head, the foundation row consisting of only two cards: me as God the mother being God, and Keith as God the father playing Satan. These two cards formed the premise from which all of my beliefs about The Game and God's Plan were derived. One day in July, I pulled out Keith's card—and the house came crashing down!

What happened is simple, really. I had been thinking long and hard about Keith and his role in my version of reality, when logic finally took over. At long last it occurred to me that there was no way God would or could consent to playing the role of Satan in The Game. Since God is love incarnate, it is not in His power to be cruel. Armed with the knowledge that Keith had volunteered to play Satan—and to target me in his cruel mind game—I came to the unmistakable conclusion that *Keith was Satan.*

For reasons I know not, I now believed there were three evil rulers of Hell: Satan, Lucifer and Max. I knew Keith was Satan, but I still had to identify the latter two. Immediately I concluded that Lucifer must be a woman and that Leah, Keith's girlfriend of long ago, was that woman.

Keith and Leah were a couple, and they visibly reigned over Hell under Max's supreme guidance. Max, the King of Hell, was so nefarious that he or she remained hidden from everyone; therefore, Max's gender, male or female, was unknown. Max existed as a voice that only Keith and Leah could hear, and these two followed Max's voice without question.

It was still up to me to find the King of Hell, Max. All of my actions were leading towards Judgment Day. I was God's main player in The Game in this world. It was all up to me. I had solved every puzzle except for the identity of Max.

Interestingly, although I believed I was God, I still prayed to God in Heaven every night. I still believed in a higher power, that there was a God above me. Far above me. And I know God heard my prayers because I am alive and well and sane again—sane enough to write this story of my insanity, sane enough to know that I never want to go to that dark place again.

Chapter 29

My mental collapse was fast and furious.

Upon deciding that Keith was evil, I logically concluded that The Game and all of its players were evil, too. I turned everything around in my mind because I now thought everything I had believed to be true was a lie. It was all a *big lie.*

I now believed that the media were not helping me to win The Game, but rather that they were trying to control me into doing what Keith, Satan, wanted me to do. And the police were not following me for my protection. On the contrary, they were stalking me to keep Keith abreast of my every move. Also, since Keith was obviously *not* in love with me, all of the songs, movies, books and television shows about Keith and me were lies. I therefore concluded that virtually every actor, musician and writer was evil. Finally, I determined that Keith had initiated all of the phone taps, bugs, eavesdropping and stalking. He had me under constant surveillance.

I went from believing that the world was composed of good, loving people who had come here to help me fulfill God's Divine Plan into believing that the world was evil. Almost everyone was on Keith's side. I was shattered.

Throughout my collapse I constantly heard voices. Carol, my guide, repeatedly told me that my thinking was correct and that she was glad that I had finally figured out Keith . . . and the rest of the world. She convinced me that there were only eight good souls in this world and that I was one of the eight. She said that it was my job to identify the remaining seven chosen ones and that once I had done so, all eight of us would find and destroy Max. This destruction of Max would occur on—would be—Judgment Day.

During both the euphoric and sad parts of my breakdown, I was obsessed with Judgment Day. I listened to the song *Solsbury Hill* by Peter Gabriel over and over and over again. I had set my CD player to repeat this one song indefinitely and am sure I must have played it for 24 hours in a row.

> *When illusion spin her net*
> *I'm never where I want to be . . .*
> *. . . I will show another me*
> *Today I don't need a replacement*
> *I'll tell them what the smile on my face meant*
> *My heart going boom, boom, boom*
> *"Hey," I said, "you can keep my things, they've come to take*
> *me home."*

> *Excerpt from song "Solsbury Hill"*
> *© 1977, Peter Brian Gabriel*
> *Real World Music Ltd.*

I dubbed this song "the song of great joy." To have written this song—to have had such glorious insight—Peter Gabriel had to be one of the chosen eight.

Then it dawned on me that the voice I was following so intently, Carol, was evil. After all, if she were good, she would have told me outright that Keith was evil. Instead, she waited for me to put it all together. A good spirit guide would help you, and Carol was no help whatsoever. With the demise of Carol's voice, new and unnamed voices immediately came to take her place. I conversed continually with these new voices until I was hospitalized.

You want to know what amazes me to this day? Throughout

the part of my breakdown I have just described, I continued to work
full time and I did my job well. But even at work, the voices never
ceased. I typed up work orders and prepared quotes while mentally
talking to my voices. I could not stop obsessing over The Game and
the identity of Max. I do not know how I managed to do all of this at
once. But I did.

Just before I was hospitalized, I was staring at my computer
at work when I thought, "Computers are evil. They are rife with
subliminal satanic messages. Satan is using computers to control
everyone."

Eureka!

Oddly, in the final days of my collapse I heard the word
"eureka" in my head about every ten seconds. That one word helped
to drive me insane. Only God knows why.

Eureka! Staring at my computer, I realized that the computer—
every computer—was the elusive Max for whom I had been searching
for so long. The unseen voice of Hell was the computer. All I had to
do now was figure out who had spearheaded the making of computers,
and I would have my Max at last!

Friday, July 30, 1993, was my last day of work. I was very
sick. I often wonder why no one at the office noticed . . .

At work that day, I thought about Max like never before. I
was determined to identify Max so that God's Plan could be fulfilled.
And I was so very sad. I needed Jesus to come back to this Earth *now*.
I needed Judgment Day so that I could escape my sorrows once and
for all. I wanted to shut off my mind. I wanted desperately to *stop
thinking,* to just *be.*

Then it came to me: Max was my father's evil twin. Yeah,
that made sense to me. Max would want to look like someone whom
he knew I loved and trusted implicitly. Next, in my weakened state—
I had been eating next to nothing and had not slept in days—I allowed
myself to imagine the worst. The very worst. What was the most
horrific notion I could imagine? Simple. My dad was Max.

I remember the energy leaving my body when I came upon
this thought. My dad . . . was Max?

And I snapped. With that one thought, I snapped.

I finished work that Friday and left. There was no going back. "My dad was Max?" I thought to myself. "But how could that be?"

Crying as I drove home, I remember thinking that I had better not let my sister Wanda see my tears. I did not want her to know that I had figured it out, that I finally knew Max's true identity.

In thinking that my dad was Max, I came to the unmistakable conclusion that the entire world was evil. Everyone but me. So I had to hide my thoughts from Wanda, for she was evil too. My mask had to be impenetrable.

When I arrived at home, I smiled at Wanda and tried to act normal. The relief I felt when she left the apartment to go to the store was immeasurable. Acting normal, at this point, was more than I could handle. But I had no choice. I needed time to think about how I would get out of this mess. Now that I knew the whole world was evil, what was to be my next step? I had to think. Think, think, think.

And all I could think to do was to pray to God to come and take me away from this world. I was so very sad, and so very afraid.

When Wanda returned to our apartment, I looked at her and thought, "That's not the same Wanda who just left."

My mind then seized upon the idea that there were three Wandas: happy Wanda, sad Wanda and angry Wanda. The three Wandas took turns living with me because they were too evil to want to be around me for any great length of time. I reasoned that it was difficult for the evil people in the world to pretend to be good and that the evil people, therefore, avoided direct contact with me as much as possible. Avoiding me was simply another part of The Game.

Of note, I believed the evil souls did not want me to know that *everyone* was evil—unless I intended to join them—because were I aware of this fact, The Game would be finished once and for all, with them the losers.

One day bled into the next. I was no longer conscious of time. While waiting for God to come and save me, I analyzed my family thoroughly. I remember thinking that Wanda was the guardian whose job it was to keep track of me night and day. My sister Julie was the hypnotist who had made me forget all the Satanists and their evil deeds. I dubbed my sister Tammy the instigator, for she had introduced me to Keith and his followers. And because she lived with Max, the true King of Hell, I concluded that my mom must be the head witch.

Still waiting for God to come and take me to Heaven, I picked up a pen and wrote out a list of every swear word I could think of, dating from olden times to today's jargon. I was daunted by the number of negative words—evil words—in existence.

I stopped eating. Out of nowhere, I believed that all food and beverages were composed of human ingredients. I had been eating bread and butter when I thought, "Butter is made from human fat." With that thought, I immediately ran into the bathroom and vomited. I starved myself for many hours before I decided that there were two food items on the market that did not contain human ingredients: cake donuts and diet cola. I went through 32 donuts and 36 colas that weekend. Oh, in my insanity I believed that the donuts had zero calories, and I dropped 8 lbs that weekend.

Just as I had obsessed over the song *Solsbury Hill*, I now played the song *The Joker*, by Steve Miller, nonstop. I kept thinking that I would be safe as long as this song kept playing. And I made sure it kept playing.

You would think that I would hate these two songs now, but I do not. They are still among my all-time favorites. For all I know, maybe something in these songs helped to bring me back to the real world. The human brain is still a mystery to me, although I like to think I have some sort of insight into mental illness.

By Sunday I was gone, gone, gone. I was completely in my own world. I decided that since I was God, it was time for me to use my innate omnipotence to confuse the Satanists. I believed that there was an ancient secret language that had been used by Satanists since the dawn of time, a language I knew. Telepathically, I began to speak to all of the Satanists simultaneously in their ancient language, and I proclaimed myself the true ruler of Hell. In my mind, the Satanists immediately followed me and my orders. The goal of their game had always been that I join them so that they could harness God's power. I was giving the people what they want, so to speak. In deposing Max, I felt that I could rest a little. Yes, declaring myself Hell's Queen seemed like a good interim plan to me. And it would have to do for now, because I needed time to devise a more permanent—and happy—solution.

The next thing I remember was looking out of my window and staring at the clouds. I saw countless evil images and became terrified anew. Then, all of a sudden, the clouds began to form words and sentences. I could see that a story was unfolding, but I was having a difficult time trying to make out all of the words. My mind kept telling me, "You've seen this before," and I then remembered having had this same vision when I was 3 years old. With renewed vigor, I stared at the words painted across the sky, and still I could not make sense of them. In the back of my mind I remembered that this story in the sky had a happy ending, a punchline really. I kept trying to read the story, the joke, but without much success. Damn! I really could have used a good laugh at this time. Ultimately, I gave up on reading the words formed by the clouds and walked away from the window.

Next, my thoughts turned towards sex. I wrote a list of every sexual word I could think of. So many things in this world relate to sex. Advertising relies on the "sex sells" premise. Fame, too, seems to be based on sexual appeal. Even in my insanity I still deemed sex a gift from God—and a pretty good gift at that—but I felt that Satanists were using sex negatively. I therefore wrote the list in an effort to better understand satanic thinking.

Late Sunday night, after Wanda had gone to bed, I analyzed my belongings. Almost unconsciously, I began to sort everything I owned into piles. When I was finished, there were five piles on my living room floor: CDs and tapes, books, jewelry, clothing and cash. I then carefully placed each pile into its own individual garbage bag. Next, I picked up the bag containing my CDs, walked out into the hallway and over to the garbage chute, and disposed of the bag and its contents. I repeated this process for each garbage bag until I came to the last bag, which contained the cash. I do not know why, but something made me hang onto the cash. I remember thinking, "Rent." Sadly, included in the jewelry pile were a gold watch and a gold ring that my two grandmothers had given to me. But as I said, I did all of this unconsciously. I believed I would be going to Heaven at any minute, so I no longer had any use for earthly goods. Oh well.

Oh well, whatever, never mind—we tend to use these words to indicate indifference; yet, in using them, we are showing that we do care. Silence is indifference. Words necessarily have meaning. (Janet trying to sound really, really deep. OK, this is self-indulgent. Oh well, whatever!)

When Wanda woke up on Monday, August 2, 1993, she noticed something was wrong. She awoke just after I had completed making an arrangement of donuts shaped like a giant "J" on my coffee table. The "J" represented Judgment Day.

Wanda then called my sister Julie, who came over right away. I was frightened beyond words. Looking from Wanda to Julie, I knew I was outnumbered and my terror grew. I tried to hide myself. I tried to pretend they were not there. For a moment, I entertained the idea that both Wanda and Julie were evil spirits, ghosts; but this notion quickly vanished. Still, though, I thought that their eyes looked blank and I prayed that they would disappear. To myself I cried, "Why won't they go away? Leave!"

In an effort to escape them, I went into Wanda's bedroom, taking with me a pen and a large pile of paper. Thankfully, my sisters did not follow me. I lay down on the floor and wrote pages and pages of notes using what I imagined was the ancient satanic script—a mishmash of lines and squiggles wherein one symbol formed an entire sentence. I did so in the hopes that I would hit upon the right spell to vanquish Wanda and Julie, to banish them from me. Still hearing Steve Miller's *The Joker* in my head and still talking to my voices, I was trying desperately to remain calm. I know I kept praying to God to help me. How was I to escape? And where would I go? After all, the whole world was evil. What was I supposed to do? "God, help me!" I prayed.

Soon after Julie had arrived at my apartment, my dad came over. Julie must have phoned him while I was in Wanda's bedroom, writing. My dad—"Max"—came into the bedroom to talk to me. *I was so scared!* In my delusional state I was seeing my dad, Ben, as Max. I saw evil glints in my dad's eyes and his fingers appeared conic, pointed. When my dad reached out to grab my arm, all I saw were the pointed fingers; so I tried my best to escape him. At some point, I lunged at him to hit him. I had decided that I was not going down without a fight. He shouted at me, "Don't you do that! I've never hit you!"

My dad was right. But I was too far gone to hear it, to believe it. Trying again to make my escape, I ran into the bathroom and attempted to bolt the door. My sister Julie managed to grab the door handle before I could lock myself in. Realizing that escape was impossible, I went back into the living room and lay down on my sofa bed, my back towards everyone. I curled up like a baby and I prayed some more. I continued to pray to God and to talk to my voices until I passed out from the medication that was later administered.

The emergency medical response team now arrived at my apartment. My dad had called for an ambulance when he realized that he could not help me. Because the ambulance workers could not legally take me to the hospital without my consent, the police were phoned; and I was apprehended under the Mental Health Act. Now the ambulance workers could take me to the hospital, where I would be certified . . . and treated.

I did not let the emergency response team take me without a fight; that is, I *tried* to fight them off. But the two emergency workers easily pinned me down and strapped me onto a gurney. The only recourse I had left open to me, the only way I could think of to keep up the fight, was my silence. I refused to talk. I refused to look at them. I remained completely unresponsive on purpose. Now in the ambulance, the female worker kept saying, "Janet, can you hear me? Do you know what's happening?"

I did not respond. I thought, "Fuck 'em! I won't give them the satisfaction of acknowledging them. If they want to kill me, fine. But I will not talk!"

I lived only five minutes away from the hospital. At some point, either in the ambulance or upon my arrival at the emergency room, I was given a shot of something. In my deluded state, I firmly believed that I had been poisoned and that I was about to die. And then, at last, I was calm. Accepting defeat—accepting my imminent death—was a release. No longer would I be afraid. Heaven awaited.

I did not die.

The next thing I remember, I was lying on a bed in a hospital room with five unfamiliar faces staring at me. My first thought was that these five doctors were robots. Then I wondered why the poison had not yet taken effect. Why was it taking so long? What did they want from me?

All of a sudden an intern leaned in towards me, and I automatically punched him . . . smack dab in the nose. I was *not* about to die meekly. In fact, I felt stronger at this moment than I had in as long as I could remember. In accepting that I was dying, all of my fears left me; all of my strength returned.

A nurse then entered my room and approached me. After I had succeeded in punching her, too, in the nose, my hands and feet were strapped to the four corners of the bed. By this time the group of five had left my room, and another female nurse had come in to watch over me, taking a seat near my bed. To myself I thought, "Satan's gloating over his victory." Whatever. I was at Heaven's doorstep. I felt fine.

Still praying, I began to feel light, like my soul was leaving my body. Thank You God! I was going to Heaven at last!

Only Heaven eluded me. Instead, I rose up to a place where I was still lying down, unable to move. I felt like I had extreme power, infinite strength, yet I could not move a muscle. And so I reasoned, "I'm in Hell. But why?"

Then I felt my soul return to my body. After struggling with my straps for about five minutes, I succeeded in freeing my left foot. I recall that the nurses on the psych ward were later mystified by my Houdini-like escape from bondage. Mercifully, I fell asleep. I had not slept since . . .

When I awoke, I saw that the same nurse was still seated in the chair by my bed. Only I was no longer afraid of her. I now knew that she was not there to hurt me.

Thank God I am logical! I reasoned that if all people were evil and had wanted me dead, I would not still be alive. However, I was not yet entirely convinced that the world was *not* evil. I now thought that there were *some* good souls in this world and that God had brought me to them. God had saved me once again. He had heard all of my prayers.

"Can I please stand up?" I asked the nurse. "My legs are sore."

"Certainly," she replied, and she freed me from the straps.

Although I did not completely trust the nurse—or anyone, for that matter—I was happy to be alive! I was returning to the real world and, man, did it feel good! My mom and dad came to see me right away. Instantly, I knew that they loved me and that none of my insanity relating to my family was real. Seeing my parents and the love evident in their eyes, I knew I would get well. I sobbed—tears of sadness mixed with tears of joy. Yes, I would return to the land of the living.

Chapter 30

Insanity is the "realm of the impossible combined with the improbable." This is my definition of insanity, anyway. The thoughts of those who are insane cannot be real, could not be real. Yet, these thoughts and ideas are very real to those who have lost the fight to remain sane. In reading about my breakdown as I have described it, you undoubtedly thought to yourself, "No way did that happen. No way."

And my reply to you: "Yeah, way!" After all, if the thoughts of an insane person seemed real, believable, these thoughts would then have to be categorized "sane."

The psychiatrist assigned to me on the hospital psych ward is the psychiatrist I see now. Without his care and perseverance, I would still be living my life in a paranoid, delusional state.

Before I discuss my medical history with this psychiatrist, I must address the fact that psychiatry is not an exact science. There is no one right pill for a given psychiatric disorder. At best, psychiatry is a process of trial and error, and the patient must understand this process and *never* lose hope. In addition, successful treatment of mental illness can be achieved only if the patient trusts the psychiatrist implicitly and follows the course of treatment prescribed by the physician without fail. Too many patients, myself included, decide to either self-medicate or quit their medications because they believe they know what is right for them. We tend to forget or ignore that a psychiatrist studies for many years to learn and practice this difficult field.

There is one amusing aspect of paranoia that became apparent to me over time. While paranoid, I would not discuss any of my delusions, hallucinations or paranoia with a psychiatrist because I feared being put away. I was paranoid of my doctors! Ironically, I had to be somewhat well before I would admit to having been sick. I do not know why, but I trusted my new psychiatrist almost immediately. Indeed, I trusted him enough to admit that I was hearing voices—an admission of extreme importance in my getting the correct meds.

The day I was admitted to the hospital, I weighed 112 lbs and my heart rate was well over 170 beats per minute. I was so weak that I could not stand up straight. Several tests were ordered including a CT scan and an EEG. I refused the latter test because I had had an EEG when I was 12 years old, and I thought it pointless to repeat the process. My heart rate and blood pressure were monitored constantly.

Initially, I was placed in a private hospital room and was restricted to remaining on the psych ward. Thank God there was a smoking room. No sooner did the nurse remove the straps that tied me to my bed than I lit up a cigarette. I managed to light up three more times before the nurses confiscated my lighter, but . . . my rebellion did gain me access to the smoking room.

When I first got up and out of bed, I brushed my teeth steadily for at least twenty minutes. I brushed my teeth so long that my lips became entirely covered in painful cold sores. I think I was trying to erase all of the bad thoughts I had envisioned by cleaning my teeth. My parents walked into my room as I was still brushing, and I was so happy to see them, I cried. As I have already said, their love for me was evident. I soon found myself thinking, "How could I ever have believed my parents, my family, were evil? What happened to me?" I determined to get well for my parents, if not for me.

I remember my mom and dad telling me repeatedly that the doctors and nurses were good people who wanted to help me get well. At first, I had my doubts. Deep down, though, I knew that my parents would not lie to me . . . and slowly I began to accept that people were good. Slowly.

At my first meeting with my psychiatrist while on the psych ward, I remember him asking me if I understood what was happening, if I understood why I was in the hospital. At this initial meeting I was wary of him, so I chose to be vague with my responses. However, within a couple of days on Largactil, an antipsychotic, I was steadily regaining my sanity; and I was trusting my doctor sufficiently to speak freely with him about my illness.

My doctor's initial diagnosis was that I was manic depressive. This diagnosis was based on both my past history and my current state. He also suspected that I might be schizoaffective. He asked me whether I could recall anything I had thought or done during the period in which I was out of it. I replied that I remembered almost everything, an admission that surprised him. Apparently, most people who return to the real world after having been in a psychotic state do not remember much about the time during which they were gone. Their insanity remains a mystery, even to them. But I did remember, like it or not.

It was the consensus of several psychiatrists that I had been catatonic when I was brought into the hospital's emergency room. When I informed my doctor that I had *chosen* not to talk to or acknowledge anyone, he was somewhat surprised. To be catatonic is to be completely in your own little world with no awareness of what is going on outside of your head. I was always fully aware—stubbornly silent, but fully aware.

At the beginning of my treatment, my psychiatrist's major concern for me was the voices, or auditory hallucinations. I kept hearing voices—voices that questioned my every thought and my every move. It felt like I had a 2-year-old living inside my brain. These voices were totally nonviolent. *Never* was I told to hurt anyone. At worst, the voices indicated that I should not trust people. Regardless, I could not make the voices go away, stop, cease.

My doctor switched me from Largactil to Haldol, a newer antipsychotic drug, on August 5, 1993. On this day, which I deem my first lucid day on the ward, I took the Haldol and bit down on it. The taste of it was awful, metallic, but I satisfied myself that the pill *was* a real drug and that the medical staff *were* trying to help me to get well. Inderal and Artane were also prescribed to combat the side effects of the Haldol (in my case, dry mouth and extreme restlessness). I remember drinking water continuously. I remember I could not sit still, not even for a minute. But my sanity was returning, and at the time that was all that really mattered to me.

Also on this day, I heard beautiful piano playing emanating from the lunchroom. I had to find out who was responsible for this wonderful sound. I went into the lunchroom where I saw a young man seated at the big old piano. His playing deeply affected me. The sound of his music filled me with happiness and hope. Many other patients had gathered in the room to hear this young man play. Music heals, pure and simple.

I introduced myself to this gifted musician. Trevor and I became friends immediately. He, too, had suffered some sort of breakdown. I did not pry. Instead, I sang while he played. The singing, the music, did much to raise my spirits. Trevor, who is close to my age, remains my friend to this day.

Trevor does not smoke. Never has. And he seldom consumes caffeinated beverages. He eats proper meals that include vegetables, fruit, meat and dairy products. And the reason I mention all of this is that a lot of people have asked me whether I think that my lifestyle choices contributed to or caused my mental illness. My response is "No." Mental illness can strike *anyone* at *any time.* Currently, there are no known ways to prevent mental illness. My psychiatrist tells me that smoking, drinking caffeinated beverages and poor diet seem to be unrelated to the illness; that is, to date studies have found no significant causative relationship between these bad habits and mental illness.

I had to leave my computer just now. It was time to take my meds. I keep my daily pills in a small, heart-shaped, silver box. Looking at my pills, I think, "There lies my life. My life is in a box."

After about a week on the ward I was moved to a regular room shared by three other ladies and me. No sooner did I lie down on my bed than the lady in the bed beside me said, "All the music is about me. All the music is my life."

Well, her remarks pissed me off no end because I knew that all of the songs in the world were about *me!*

This lady then informed me that she was Mary Magdalene and that Judgment Day was at hand.

To myself I thought, "She's completely deluded! I'm Jesus, so I would know if she were Mary!"

After this discussion, I did my best to avoid the "crazy" people on the ward. Of course, all of this is funny to me now, but at the time I really thought that I was normal and that, yes, I was God. Even when my psychiatrist questioned me about the Jesus thing—nurses had informed him that I was telling other patients my "true" identity—I told him with absolute conviction that I was, indeed, Jesus.

Delusions of grandeur are extremely common among manics. I came upon this knowledge after having met many manic patients. Most of us who suffer from mental illness think we were or are some famous biblical personage. But in my thinking that I was God, I was alone. None of the other patients I met imagined themselves to be God. Just me. And I think I know why. I have always striven for perfection in everything I do; therefore, for me to have a delusion of grandeur that was truly grand, who else could I be but God? Strangely, believing myself to be the all-loving deity helped me to get well. As God, I feared no one and forgave everyone. Also, as God, I loved everyone and believed the world was full of good, loving people. Go figure.

Nearing the end of my stay on the psych ward, my psychiatrist asked me whether I still believed myself to be Jesus or God. I answered honestly that I now considered myself God's star child. When I asked my doctor if this was OK, he said, "Yes."

I was on the psych ward from August 2 to August 17, 1993. During that time my family visited me every day, and I soon realized that I was the lucky one. For you see, I noticed that the majority of the patients on the ward had few or no visitors. I do not know whether the absence of visitors was due to fear of this "silent" illness or due to the mistaken notion that mental illness is not a *real* illness. Regardless, it was disheartening to see that so many mentally ill patients were on their own, alone.

My discharge meds included Haldol, Inderal and Artane.

Who comes up with these names? Hi, I'm Janet from the city of Clozaril on the planet Zoloft. Our national flower is the beautiful Haloperidol, and our national bird is the majestic Largactil.

Upon leaving the hospital, I felt literally reborn. God had restored my mind and my life. As my doctor wrote in my discharge summary, I was "like a child, wide-eyed with fascination with the world." Everything felt new to me. Everything gave me joy. I continued to see my psychiatrist weekly so that he could monitor my progress. I knew I was in good hands.

Once back at home in my apartment, my mom urged me to take martial arts lessons again. The breakdown had taken such a physical toll on my body that I had to do something to rebuild my strength. Following my mom's sage advice, I signed up for tae kwon do lessons right away. Before I began my lessons, I had a talk with my instructor to whom I disclosed my illness and my current lack of physical strength. The instructor was very compassionate. He told me to do the best that I could and to sit down and rest as needed.

At first I was physically unable to complete even the warm-up exercises. It took a good month before I was able to keep up with the rest of the class. In that time I regained some of the weight I had lost and was back to 120 lbs. I stuck with the tae kwon do lessons long enough to earn my yellow belt and to break a wooden board with my foot, something I had wanted to do since I was a young child. Breaking the board was a signal to me that I was strong again, so I stopped my lessons. Besides, I was worried about breaking a finger and not being able to play my guitar. Guitar comes first. Always.

My psychiatrist felt it would be several months before I would be well enough to work again. I therefore applied for unemployment insurance and tried to subsist on that income as best I could. Even had I wished to continue my tae kwon do lessons, I simply did not have the money for such luxuries.

I was definitely still sick. The mania in the form of extreme energy continued, and I still heard voices. These auditory hallucinations, however, mainly came out at night. As soon as my head hit the pillow, I would hear voices. In an attempt to dispel these nocturnal voices, I began leaving my radio on at bedtime. Focusing on the music helped to rid me of some of the voices.

I should note that I made one major lifestyle change upon leaving the hospital: I cut out caffeine, allowing myself only two mugs of coffee per day. Given the mania, I had to concede that coffee was not a good idea at this time. Furthermore, while I was in the hospital, a physician had strongly urged that I abstain from caffeine altogether. This physician was very concerned about my rapid heart rate. Although giving up my coffee was somewhat akin to giving up breathing, I followed the doctor's orders. I *really* wanted to get well. As for my cigarette consumption . . .

I'm an imperfect person in an imperfect world. I used to argue in favor of tobacco by saying that it is a substance that exists in nature. God put tobacco on this planet. But deep down, I don't believe God thought that we would take this plant, dry it out and smoke it! It's rather absurd, isn't it?

. . . I always go back to my cigarettes. I cannot decide whether the stress of quitting smoking would be better or worse than the stress I feel over the health risks of smoking. Rock—me—hard place.

By the end of August my psychiatrist added Tegretol to my meds to act as a mood stabilizer. He was still very concerned about my auditory hallucinations, but I assured him that I was improving in that the voices seemed to be diminishing. My restlessness, however, continued.

"Auditory hallucinations." I love it! Such a fancy way of saying "voices."

As I was never much good at doing nothing, I decided to take on something new, something completely different. Accordingly, I signed up for a night school chemistry class. My lack of scientific knowledge had always made me feel somewhat inadequate—while in high school I had studied only biology—so I felt it was time to remedy the situation. More importantly, I wanted to see if my brain was still functioning as well as it had in the past, prior to my breakdown. I am perfectly serious here. I truly wondered whether my ability to memorize things and to be logical had suffered as a result of my mental illness. Well, I averaged around 97% on my chemistry tests and felt completely reassured that my brain still worked as it had. Studying chemistry rekindled my interest in the subject of God and creation. Once again I began to obsess over the topic of God. And I continued to be manic.

I found myself wondering, "What did God do *before* He created the universe?" The idea that God was lazy was preposterous, so I came upon the notion that God had been sleeping. His sleep was akin to being in a coma. I felt that He was stuck in His line of thought. Specifically, I believed He was perpetually thinking about the past. And since God's past is infinite, He could remain thinking backward forever, without end. I call this stage of God's existence "the big sleep."

What happened next is obvious. God realized His past was infinite, and He awoke. My contention is that God looped time so that He could begin to move forward. To achieve this loop, He merely had to rethink a previous thought. That done, He and time could now move infinitely forward.

I next wondered, "What was God's first thought?" I instantly concluded that it had to be "I." One has to proclaim, acknowledge, oneself to begin to *think.* I had the notion that God's first thoughts went as follows:

> *I*
> *I think*
> *I think "I"*
> *I think, "I think . . ."*
> *I know*
> *I know "I"*
> *I know "I think"*
> *I know "I think 'I' "*
> *I THINK THEREFORE I AM.*

One has to acknowledge one's *existence* to begin to *live!* Interestingly, in the Old Testament God refers to Himself as "I AM." I guess when I studied the Bible in university, this statement stayed with me. Whatever. I remember that I was very pleased with this theory—I still am.

I have many more theories on God and creation. Perhaps these theories will be a book unto themselves one day. However, I cannot leave this topic without addressing my love for the color black.

If you take every color in existence and blend them all together, the resulting color is black—gray, if white is the last color added. So I think black is the color of colors and is, therefore, a highly positive color. (Gray, as far as I am concerned, is actually light black.) Furthermore, I deem black, ultra-dark blue. As such, black is my two favorite colors in one. Now, if you look at a light and shut your eyes, you will see scarlet red. Possibly, my hatred of red stems from my belief that red is the color you see when you close your eyes to the light.

All right. I will concede that red could be viewed positively as being the light one sees in the darkness—the light that remains with you even if you choose to shut out the light—but this concession does not alter my hatred of red! I can tolerate blue-red and maroon, but scarlet red, aargh!

These God Theories are the product of mania, and I thoroughly love this aspect of my mania. I continue to hold onto the hope that I will one day write a book that logically proves God's existence. But I have a lot more thinking to do—a veritable plethora of ideas to consider—before I will get there.

Yeah! I've always wanted to use the phrase "veritable plethora" in real life. Enough self-indulgence.

In September 1993 I discussed some of my God Theories with my psychiatrist. He immediately reasoned that I was in a manic phase and suggested that I try Lithium, as it is the drug of choice for the treatment of manic depression. For me, it was anathema. I found myself sobbing continually while I was on this drug. Given my adverse reaction to Lithium, my doctor told me to cease taking this drug. I went back on Haldol and Tegretol and remained on these two meds until January 1994.

Also in September, I tried to rekindle my relationship with Brendan. I did, for a while. We split up once and for all in November 1993, but not before he had managed to hurt me beyond words. He told me to "Get a life." Because of this unfeeling remark and because I was particularly vulnerable at this time, I fell into a depression that November that stayed with me for a very long time. I forced myself to finish my night school class, which was quite difficult under the circumstances—I have already noted that depression renders one fatigued, uninspired—and I did my best to appear and be happy. But the idea that I was alone again, and would probably remain so, made me sad. Very sad. It certainly did nothing to further my recovery.

I cannot emphasize this enough: people are afraid of mental illness and are, therefore, afraid to be around those who are mentally ill. If this book promotes better understanding of the illness, I will have succeeded in my goal. Here is a thought I had years ago that has stayed with me:

Alone in my thoughts, I see little of you
Or what your world means to me.

I hope everyone will try to understand my world, rather than fear it. I hope.

Chapter 31

It took many years for me to lose my mind, and it took a couple of years before my psychiatrist found the right combination of meds to heal me, to correct my chemical imbalance. My doctor's hands, however, were tied during this recovery period because I could not afford to take the drugs that he recommended—and that I required. By January 1994 I was forced to discontinue taking Haldol altogether. My budget would not permit this newer and more effective medication. In its stead, I returned to Largactil, combined with Tegretol, for the treatment of my imbalance.

I am *not* knocking Largactil, also known as Thorazine. Largactil was the first successful antipsychotic made, and it did work for me. It prevented me from succumbing to the bad thoughts I had suffered and it kept me in the real world. But Largactil did not work ideally. Although I could function under this drug, the nocturnal voices persisted and I was exhausted most of the time. By April I was forced to quit my chemistry course as a direct result of my terrible mood swings and extreme fatigue.

My moods were highly unstable; that is, my mood could change from one minute to the next. I could go from extreme mania to severe depression in the blink of an eye. As such, it was not the easiest condition to treat—or to live with, for that matter. Thankfully, neither my psychiatrist nor I gave up the fight.

In May 1994 my unemployment insurance ran out, and I was forced to look for work again. I was not well; I knew I was still sick. But I could not afford to live on welfare. I had to pay rent, I had to eat, and I had to buy my meds. I therefore began my job hunt in April, just prior to the cessation of my unemployment insurance coverage.

I phoned *every* business in the Yellow Pages that might have a clerical position. I found nothing. My sporadic job history was working against me, and I dared not disclose that I had left my previous position due to mental illness. At the end of April I got lucky. A friend of mine, whom I had met through Brendan, told me that a secretarial position had just become vacant at his place of work. I applied for this job immediately. Based on my work history, my education and my friend's recommendation, I was hired the next day. The relief I felt was enormous. I would be able to pay my bills—for a while, anyhow. Deep down, I suspected that I would not last long in this job. My illness was too severe at this time.

And I was correct. I was not yet ready to work, a fact that became evident within a week of my starting at this new job. I had been hired as a production coordinator/order desk clerk. This position differed from my previous clerical jobs in that I was continually on the phone taking orders. My past positions did not involve telephone work. I just typed. Now I had to take telephone orders, do data entry of production records, track shipments, schedule production and file. Had I been well, I am sure that I could have handled this multi-task position. My employer and coworkers were great! But . . .

I left work each day feeling completely stressed out. Once home, I would fall asleep for a couple of hours, wake up to watch the television for an hour or so, and then go to bed by 9:00 p.m. That I was exhausted all of the time is an understatement. I could not even enjoy my weekends. The exhaustion rendered me immobile. I would sleep all of Saturday and most of Sunday. No sooner did I begin to feel awake than the cycle started over again.

Ultimately, I fell into a deep depression, the worst I had ever known: I fell into *despair*. This was a sadness that I could not shake off, as I had done so many times before. With despair, I was too tired to fight off the sadness; and, to me, that *is* despair—being too weak to fight off your depression. I had just been notified of a pay raise when I crashed.

My depression became severe enough that my psychiatrist advised me to go back onto the psych ward. He was concerned that I might attempt suicide, and rightfully so.

Although part of my depression related to my single status, the greater part of it grew out of the voices and a new disorder: obsessive-compulsive disorder, OCD. I was repeatedly hearing voices saying things like "that bitch" or "that bastard." Every time I talked to someone in person or on the telephone and said or heard the word "goodbye," I would hear the word "bitch" or "bastard" as a loud whisper in my right ear (my voices always spoke into my right ear). Another phrase that I heard over and over was "If thine eye offends thee, pluck it out," a phrase that terrified me, as I took it quite literally. These repetitious voices, usually triggered by some word or phrase, fell into the category of OCD.

The worst of my OCD-related voices were those saying, "God damn . . ." The ellipses included "God," "Jesus," "The Church," and so on. These auditory hallucinations were so hard on me that I phoned a Catholic priest to explain my voices to him and to seek forgiveness. The priest was very compassionate and informed me that God understands my illness and that there was nothing to forgive, as I was not responsible for my voices. Even though I felt somewhat better after this conversation, this reassurance, what I really wanted— needed—was for the voices to stop once and for all.

Following my psychiatrist's advice, I returned to the hospital psych ward on July 4, 1994, and remained there for eight days. While I was on the ward, my psychiatrist advised me to remain on Fluanxol, an antipsychotic drug that I had been taking since May 25, 1994, and to start taking Zoloft, an antidepressant. In May, my doctor had eliminated Tegretol from my list of meds because it seemed to be doing nothing for me. By this time I was officially diagnosed as both manic depressive and obsessive compulsive.

I couldn't just settle for one psychiatric disorder? I feel so greedy. I can make light of it now, but at the time my sorrow seemed infinite.

When I left the psych ward, I did so under my psychiatrist's recommendation that I not work, at least for the remainder of July.

Once home again, I decided to get a kitten. I wanted someone to love, and I had always had an affinity for cats. I found the most affectionate cat in the world. A cat named "Boo." I named him River to begin with, but one day I looked at him and said, "Hey there, Boo," and the name stuck. I firmly believe that pets do improve your mood, your outlook. I guess it is the unconditional love thing. Whatever. Boo, or BooBoo, always makes me smile.

I was fortunate in that I had saved up enough money to remain at home for the remainder of July. However, I knew I would have no choice but to seek employment come August. And I got lucky once more. I applied for a job with the housing industry company for whom I had worked just prior to the Big Breakdown of 1993, and they hired me back. Indeed, they hired me with full knowledge of my illness, indicating that my position would be *mainly* part time. I deemed this situation ideal for I felt that I could handle the stress of a part-time position and that the occasional eight-hour day would not be too hard on me.

Upon returning to work, I became manic . . . again. Between August and October 1994, I got seven tattoos, each with its own special meaning. (While manic, I had gotten one tattoo in 1989 of a G clef and heart-shaped notes.) My first tattoo at this time was of the archangel Gabriel, which I had placed upon my left shoulder. I felt that this angel would bring me good luck and would protect me from evil. And Gabriel, with his horn, is the musical angel in my eyes. Next, I got a tattoo of the "blue bird of happiness," as I call it, on my thigh. But my favorite of all my tattoos is the band of blue lilies that I had tattooed around my upper left arm, like a bracelet. I think of this tattoo as a promise ring that I will one day find my true soulmate.

I was about to get a nose piercing when my mom intervened. I find this story quite amusing. I was in the tattoo parlor awaiting my piercing, when my mom phoned to speak to the artist who was about to do the piercing. I guess she explained to him that I was in a manic phase and that under no circumstances should he give me the piercing

I had requested. When this big, burly, somewhat scary-looking gentleman got off the phone, he said simply, "That was your mother. I can make you a clip-on nose ring. That's the best I can do. Sorry."

A week later, I bought a silver clip-on nose ring that I sported for no more than a couple of months. Today, I am very thankful that my mom intervened. At the rate I was going, I would have been covered in tattoos and punched full of holes. Scary.

What my job was supposed to be and what it was were two different things.

Well that's no big surprise.

From the day I started back to work, I was putting in eight-hour days, Monday through Friday. When I asked what had happened to the part-time hours that I had been promised, my employer said that they would come in time. I did not *have* time. The stress of my job rapidly became too great for me. Not only was I working full-time hours, but I was also doing the work of two people once more. By the end of September the manic trip I had been enjoying ended abruptly, and I was back in the abyss of despair.

On October 4, 1994, I went to see The Rolling Stones in concert—in Edmonton—but I was too sad to focus on it, to enjoy it. This concert was my dream come true, but the thrill of it was lost to me due to my illness.

On Wednesday, October 5, 1994, my doctor advised that I return to the psych ward. I checked myself onto the ward that same day. At this point I was diagnosed as being a "rapid cycler," a person who suffers from four or more manic and/or depressive episodes within a one-year period. Hoping that Lithium would solve my problems, I asked my doctor if I could try this drug again; but it failed just as badly as it had during my first trial. So my psychiatrist decided to keep me on the Fluanxol, Zoloft and Largactil, but in different doses.

At this juncture, or perhaps a little earlier, my psychiatrist recommended Clozaril, a high-end antipsychotic. Although Clozaril is used primarily in the treatment of schizophrenia, my doctor informed me that this drug was proving successful in the treatment of manic depression as well. But Clozaril has one major drawback in that it requires weekly or biweekly blood tests to monitor the white blood cell count. Because of this drawback, I refused the drug. Regardless of this drawback, I could not *afford* the drug.

I remained on the psych ward until October 19, 1994. When I contacted my employer, I discovered that they no longer required my services. No surprise there. Unemployment insurance beckoned me anew.

On Thursday, October 27, 1994—a week after leaving the ward—I decided suicide was the only answer to my troubles, my sadness. I had just tried dating for the first time since Brendan. The man in question seemed very interested in me, but there was one small problem: he already had a girlfriend. He insisted, however, that he truly cared for me and that he was torn between his longtime girlfriend and me. In short, he chose her. And I chose to overdose. But this man was *not* the cause of my suicide attempt. He just came into my life at the wrong time. It was my constant sadness coupled with my single status that led me to this final solution. I was sick of feeling sad all the time, and I was *really* sick of being single. I felt that life without a true love, a soulmate, was not worth living. So, that night I swallowed forty Largactil tablets, grabbed my Bible and lay down on my bed to die. I should say that my sister Wanda, my roommate, was out of town on this date.

I quickly discovered that it is impossible to kill yourself with a Bible in your hands. At least that was the case with me. Within seconds of lying down on my bed, I changed my mind. I got up, hurried to the telephone and dialed my parents' number; but their phone was busy. Beginning to panic, I phoned a friend of mine. He said he was on his way, but I knew that the drive from his place to mine took about twenty minutes. Growing more anxious, I then called the operator, explained the emergency and asked her to put my call through to my parents' line.

She did. I told my parents what I had done. My friend and my parents arrived at my apartment at the same time. Somehow my friend had managed to complete the drive to my place in ten minutes, and I am grateful to him to this day for his caring.

As it was the closest hospital to my home, my parents sped me to the ER located at the same hospital where I had received psychiatric treatment. My psychiatrist came to see me as quickly as he could. He walked into my cubicle wherein he found me hooked up to several monitors. Looking at him, I felt that I had let him down. The first thing I said to him was, "Can I have a cigarette now?"

My doctor agreed to my request. I had to remain on the psych ward overnight as a precaution so that my health could be monitored. When I talked to my psychiatrist the following morning, I assured him that I would *never* again attempt suicide, that I had learned my lesson. He then allowed me to go home.

Ironically, in attempting to die, I discovered just how much I wanted to live. And live I did.

I left the hospital that day with a new, positive outlook on life. And slowly, my mania returned. I started to write songs again, something I had not done in years. Over the next two months I wrote at least 50 songs. I also began to spend money like there was no tomorrow, and I maxed out my credit card in the process.

Yes, I was definitely manic, and the mania was growing daily. By December I was full-blown manic. The ecstasy was wonderful, while it lasted . . .

In December, I started to hang out at The Watering Hole again, a place I had not visited in ages. Not a good sign. I also began to revisit the terrible delusions I had suffered during my Big Breakdown of 1993. Once again I was believing that the world—my family included—was evil and that I was being followed. Nightmarish visions in which I had been abused plagued me anew. Ultimately, I believed I was God.

I was extremely lucky that this third breakdown was stopped before it could reach the terrible proportions of the Big Breakdown. This time my family knew the signs. This time my family knew what to do. My mom has told me on numerous occasions that when I am deeply manic, my face changes. I have photographs wherein the changes are obvious. My mom, therefore, could tell just by looking at me that I was sick again.

My dad brought me to the hospital ER on Friday, December 23, 1994. He tricked me into going with him by telling me that I was merely going there to "talk to a psychiatrist." After the talk, I left the hospital, walked home and went to bed. That this chat was about having me committed did not register with me . . . so I left.

My dad came to my apartment the next morning and returned me to the psych ward where I was officially committed. My pulse at this time was over 200 beats per minute. Immediately, I was given a sedative. My heart rate and blood pressure were monitored every hour. Even when I finally fell asleep, my pulse was high—170 beats per minute—but by the following morning, it had returned to a more normal rate.

Because it was Christmas day, my psychiatrist permitted me to go home and have Christmas dinner with my family on the condition that I would return to the ward by 9:00 p.m. I was ecstatic that I was able to celebrate the holiday with my family. The bad thoughts I had been having regarding my family had disappeared. I knew they loved me. I knew I loved them.

When I returned to the ward, I brought a guitar with me. I played and sang for everyone there. The music helped me and the other patients feel better. As always, music gave me hope.

At long last, I decided it was time to follow my doctor's advice: I agreed to try Clozaril, the drug he had been recommending for so long. On January 6, 1995, after a few days on no medication, I began taking Clozaril . . . and have been on this drug ever since.

When I first took Clozaril, a weekly blood test to monitor the white blood cell count was required. And my initial aversion to taking Clozaril stemmed directly from this aspect of the drug. Not that I was afraid of needles; rather, I was opposed to the inconvenience of having to go to a laboratory all the time. Furthermore, assuming the Clozaril did work for me, I had no idea how I was going to pay for this drug once I was out of the hospital.

AISH: Assured Income for the Severely Handicapped. A girl I met on the psych ward suggested that I apply for AISH. I spoke to my psychiatrist about this program, and he agreed that my illness was severe enough to warrant my going on AISH. Time and time again, I had tried to work and I had gotten sick. My doctor therefore agreed that I was unable to work—that my illness was such that I could not work. With the help of a hospital social worker, I applied for and was awarded AISH, which includes full coverage of prescription drugs. I could now remain on Clozaril . . . and I *needed* to remain on Clozaril. Without this miracle drug, I would have spent my life on and off the psych ward.

Clozaril worked for me as no other drug had done. Within a couple of months my auditory hallucinations—with the exception of OCD-related voices—disappeared, as did both my paranoia and my delusions. In six months' time I was semi-normal. After a year had passed, I was sane. This new sanity was something I had not experienced since my early childhood years. This new sanity was and is wonderful!

Chapter 32

I left the psych ward on January 13, 1995. The only medication I was taking when discharged was Clozaril.

While still on the ward, I decided that I was going to make a new tape of my music because I was not entirely happy with the demo tape I had recorded in 1991. Besides, I liked my newer music. My words and melodies had improved over the years. Accordingly, as soon as I left the hospital I rented a 4-track recorder, and I looked up an old friend who knew a lot about recording, producing and mixing. With his advice in mind, I set about making my first album.

"Album," for those of you born after the advent of CDs, is the word we old fogies used in ancient times when only record players and tape recorders existed for the enjoyment of music.

Playing all of the instruments—rhythm guitar, lead guitar and drums—and singing, I recorded 11 of my songs. I was very fortunate in that I convinced another old friend to play lead guitar for me on three of the tracks. The first friend I mentioned, the producer, professionally mixed my homemade tape, which I named *Fire One*. Upon finishing my album, I was quite pleased with myself because I had actually followed up on one of my manic plans.

When manic you have so many ideas, so many planned undertakings, that often the end result is that you accomplish, or finish, nothing. I have many half-written songs that can attest to this aspect of mania. Indeed, throughout my life I have quit while in the middle of many projects because of either mania or depression.

Under the high dose of Clozaril that I was initially prescribed, I slept for 12 to 16 hours a day. Even in my waking hours, I was perpetually tired. But you know what? The pleasure and joy of being *sane*, at long last, more than made up for the fatigue.

Music became my passion again. And for the first time I could remember, I did not mind being single . . . unmarried . . . a spinster. I was finally able to enjoy the many gifts God has bestowed upon me. I finally decided to *take life as it comes*, advice my mom had given me countless times over the years. I wrote a little prayer recently that calls to mind this advice and that helps me to remain happy.

> *Whatever happens*
> *So shall it be*
> *For I will to do God's will*
> *And thus I am free.*

> *Poem "Freedom" © 2001, J. M. Knudsen*

Obviously my strong faith in God has contributed to my wellness. But there is one thing in particular that helped me to heal: the guitar.

In the summer of 1995 I busked at a local farmers' market on weekends. I loved being able to play and sing for an audience again. It had been so long, too long. That summer I made a crucial decision: I resolved to learn classical guitar; I resolved to *master* the guitar.

While working at the music store back in the '80s, I had tried to teach myself classical guitar by studying method books. However, my inability to play well at the higher levels indicated to me that something was lacking in my technique, a shortcoming that bothered me no end. I could not and would not accept that I was unable to play. Rather, I knew that I could play any song if taught properly. I therefore phoned the local music teachers association and asked whom they would recommend as a classical guitar teacher. Their answer was instantaneous: Carl Lotsberg.

I phoned Carl that same day and we discussed my situation. I explained to him that I had tried to teach myself classical guitar in the past but that I knew my technique was not right. Carl laid down the law. He said that he would probably have to start me at a remedial level in order to undo the damage I had done in teaching myself.

Remedial! That was a hard pill to swallow, but . . . deep down I knew Carl was right. I resolved to do whatever was required in order to master the guitar. Informing Carl that I was fully prepared to follow his lead, I began my lessons in October 1995.

At first, I practiced for approximately thirty minutes a day. My attention span was limited by the fatigue and inability to concentrate that accompanied my being on Clozaril. Despite these negative side effects, I learned quickly. Over time, my practice sessions increased in duration. I went from playing at a remedial level to completing Grade 3 of The Royal Conservatory of Music method in my first year of lessons. And I discovered something new and wonderful about music, something I had suspected all along but could not prove—music heals.

The discipline of classical guitar—reading music, scales, technique exercises—accompanied by the beauty of the music itself, proved therapeutic. I believe it was the combination of my meds *and* my music that ultimately healed me, that healed my body *and* soul. My psychiatrist agrees.

When I play classical guitar, my mind is completely enthralled. There is no room to feel or to think about anything other than the music. Playing classical guitar most definitely helped to eliminate the voices that had plagued me for so long. And due to its meditative quality, the guitar helped to quell my mania. Lastly, playing classical guitar gave and continues to give me joy and a sense of accomplishment. Playing this beautiful instrument helped to eradicate the depression and despair I had lived with since childhood.

I feel especially blessed to have found such a wonderful guitar teacher! It is one thing to play an instrument well, but to teach well is an art unto itself. To be a mentor truly is the highest form of giving, and so I am grateful that Carl Lotsberg chose to be a music teacher.

My OCD-related voices disappeared by 1996. Unfortunately, three new obsessions came into my life to take their place. I became obsessed with fire and could not leave my apartment without first checking all of the ashtrays and appliances ten times or more. I developed a strange obsession with my car. Whenever I drove somewhere, I repeatedly had to check to ensure that all of the car doors were locked and that the car was in park. Often I would park my car, walk away from it and then feel forced to return to it to check it all over again. My final obsession related to my guitar. Whenever I went to my music lessons, I would place my guitar in the trunk of my car. I would then feel compelled to open and close the trunk three or more times—and then open and close my guitar case a few times—before I would feel satisfied that the instrument was, in fact, safely in the trunk. Many times, after having driven no more than a block, I would feel compelled to pull over, park the car and repeat this ritual checking of my trunk and my guitar.

My psychiatrist prescribed Zoloft to combat these obsessive behaviors. He informed me that my OCD could be a side effect of the Clozaril. Just my luck. The drug that had restored my sanity was now driving me insane! Thankfully, the Zoloft worked as desired, and the only OCD behavior that remains with me today is the occasional intrusive auditory hallucination. I can live with that. I am sufficiently well that these negative voices no longer hurt me as they did in the past. In taking these voices for what they are—uncontrollable events of no significance—I have curtailed them for the most part.

In addition to studying the guitar, I found two other hobbies that proved meditative: needlepoint and knitting. I have designed many sweaters and dresses in recent years. On my budget, I almost have to make my own clothes. But I do enjoy creativity. I believe God gave us the gift of creativity so that we could have an inkling of what it is like to be Him. Just a thought.

The cigarettes . . . have become a source of anxiety for me. Although I have never suffered from any smoking-related illnesses, I worry about the possibility of one day becoming sick as a direct result of my smoking. Worse, I worry about the second-hand smoke I emit around my sister Wanda and my parents, all of whom quit smoking many years ago. The one time I tried to go without cigarettes was in July 1993, right smack dab in the middle of the Big Breakdown. I was smoke free for ten long days. Basically, I had to be completely off my nut to succeed in quitting this vice. I currently blame the stress of writing this book as the cause of my continued smoking. But I know that I will always find another cause, another reason, not to quit. That is easy enough to do. However, now that I am sane and happy, I find that I can no longer justify my habit to myself. In other words, I do not believe me. My excuses are lame and I know it.

And I bring up the subject of cigarettes again because I believe that they play a major role in the final mental disorder from which I have suffered since May 1996—anxiety attacks.

Anxiety attacks are horrible. While in the throes of these attacks, you feel like you cannot breathe, like you are going to pass out, like you are going to die. I had one or two such attacks in 1996; however, the attacks became almost a daily event within a year from their inception.

In May 1997 my psychiatrist added Ativan to my list of meds in order to combat the anxiety attacks. And I have been on what I dub "the magic three"—Clozaril, Zoloft and Ativan—ever since. These three drugs in the right doses have given me back my life. And it is a good life! I still sleep 12 to 14 hours a day. I still have the occasional intrusive auditory hallucination. Once in a blue moon I have an anxiety attack. However, for the most part, I am *well.* I am *happy*!

I remain on assistance, AISH, because my illness impedes the likelihood of my being able to handle the stress of a job. My psychiatrist believes that working would more than likely precipitate another breakdown. I do not know what tomorrow holds in store. But I do know that I look forward to my tomorrows now that I am well.

In October 1997 I saw The Rolling Stones in concert, in Edmonton, again. This time I was well and was therefore able to enjoy the show fully. My dream came true . . . twice.

In February 1998 I had the honor of playing guitar at my sister Julie's wedding. It was a wonderful experience for me as it was my

New Power

first public performance playing classical guitar. Many of the guests later told me how much they had enjoyed my playing. Me, I was happy that I had been able to give my sister the greatest gift I have to offer—my music.

I should make it clear that I am still studying the guitar and have now reached the Grade 10 level of The Royal Conservatory of Music method. In 1998 I went for the Grade 3 Conservatory test, and I won the first place medal for that grade level. In spring of 2000 I played at a local music festival and won first place in the adult contemporary category, playing at a ninth grade level.

And all was well with the world . . .

I had a mini-breakdown in February 2001. It was a manic-depressive breakdown complete with visual hallucinations, delusions and paranoia. I do not know what triggered this episode, as I had been well since January 1995. What I do know is that I became extremely manic for about a week, and then I became terribly depressed—depressed to the extreme that I could not stand up straight. Once again I was thinking that my sister Wanda was evil, because I was seeing evil glints in her eyes. Once again I was questioning whether my parents were evil, too.

Because of my past experience with the illness, I knew how to read the signs. I confessed to my mom the thoughts that were going through my head, and she immediately took me to the ER. Because my doctor knew that I was aware of my illness, and also because I did not want to return to the psych ward, he treated me as an outpatient for a week. He doubled my dosage of Clozaril, which had been reduced over the years, and increased my dosage of Ativan. Within a month or so, I was back to normal. Well.

It was this final breakdown that inspired me to write my story. I had considered doing so in the past, but only fleetingly. I now believe God gave me this mini-lapse to inspire me to write. I think my story needed to be told in order to bring about a greater understanding of mental illness. As I said at the start of this book, I am in the unique position of remembering what happened—what I thought and did—throughout my illness.

So there you have it. Except . . .

Afterword

I have spent a great deal of time pondering mental illness. Psychiatrists say that it stems from chemical imbalances and are correct in their assertions. But still, I wonder whether mental illness—that is, the thoughts of those who are mentally ill—can be more fully explained. I have a few theories that I have developed based upon my experience, theories that may apply to other mentally ill people.

We all dream. We all know that we forget many of our dreams. I am certain that everyone has had the experience of waking up from a nightmare and not remembering what that nightmare was about.

I believe many of my psychotic thoughts were the products of remembered nightmares. The first time I would have a bad dream, that was what it was—a bad dream. But when I had this *same* dream twenty years later, the dream now had the quality of being a *memory*. Because I could not remember that the dream *was* a dream to begin with, the dream became a memory only, a very real memory. So dreams became reality.

Where did the nightmarish visions come from? My contention is that they were a combination of reality and extreme empathy. For example, when I watched television as a young child, I would often hear news reports about missing children, abused children, body parts being found in garbage dumpsters, rape, pornography . . . sadly, this list could go on. In my nightmares, I would then become the victim of these atrocities; I would experience the pain and fear and trauma personally. So now, not only did my nightmares *seem* real as memories, but they also *felt* real due to empathy.

That our brains have perfect memory is integral to my theory. Consciously or subconsciously, we *do* remember everything we see, hear, experience and dream.

It was not until I got well that I realized many of my psychotic thoughts were actually nightmares of long ago, because I could now remember quite vividly when I had had a given dream for the first time. And I was plagued by the idea that I had been the victim in my dreams until I seized upon the concept of extreme empathy.

To summarize, my first theory is that some psychotic thoughts are the combination of dreams, perfect memory and extreme empathy. Your nightmares become your reality.

Next, I pondered my paranoia. Why did I believe I was being followed, tapped, bugged and eavesdropped upon?

Although my answer is unscientific, it is the only answer that I have come upon that makes sense: I have psychic abilities. Here are some real-life examples of these abilities that surprised me as much as anyone when they occurred.

In 1999 I had a nightmare in which I was 3 years old. In this nightmare, some cloaked figure had severed my head from my body. I then saw myself in a taxicab holding my severed head in my hands. Looking at the cab driver, I discovered that David Bowie was behind the wheel. He quickly drove me to the hospital where my head was reattached to my body.

What a crazy dream!

When I had my mini-breakdown in February 2001, my mom called a cab to take me to the hospital ER. I sat down on the passenger seat of the cab, crying. When I looked at the driver, I was shocked to discover that he was the spitting image of David Bowie. My mom, who was with me in the cab, can attest to this fact. I asked my driver whether anyone had ever told him that he looked like Bowie. He replied, "All the time."

The psychic metaphor here is obvious. I lost my head (breakdown) as a child (I went to the ER with my mom) and "David Bowie" (the cab driver) drove me to the ER where I was treated (head now reattached to body).

Another example of a psychic dream relates to The Watering Hole, the bar I frequented so much while I was very ill. Starting in January 2000, I began to have a recurring dream in which I would go to The Hole—only in this dream the bar had changed dramatically. It had doubled or tripled in size. This dream made no sense to me because the property, land, required to enlarge the bar did not exist.

In February 2001 I went back to The Hole for the first time in five years. I walked into the lounge area and, lo and behold, the lounge had now doubled in size. A nearby building had been torn down thus enabling this expansion to take place.

One more quick example. For years I had a recurring nightmare in which I was swimming in a muddy swamp with all manner of scary creatures floating around me. The swamp, however, was like a swimming pool, and there was nothing to stop me from getting out of this pool. But I did not get out—I wanted out badly—but I did not get out.

This nightmare has stopped. When I ceased hanging around Keith and his crowd, I escaped the swamp once and for all.

I am not limited to having psychic dreams. I am unusually psychic in other areas as well.

Over the years, I have been very much aware that my fashions are followed. By this I mean that my favorite pieces of clothing, jewelry and accessories seem to become the trend about a year after I have sported them. For example, a trend that I began in 1989 has now been adopted. When I went out to clubs or bars back then, I always wore a plain, silver ring on my right-hand little finger that I dubbed my "single ring." Just as married couples have wedding rings, I had my single ring. Recently, I saw a girl on the news who was trying to market her new idea—the "single ring." According to this girl, her rings were to be worn on the same finger that I had designated so long ago. I was annoyed that my idea had been "stolen."

The numbers I talked about in my story are another psychic phenomenon. As I explained, if I felt the number was 2, I would see 2s everywhere. Right now, I see the number 32 all of the time. Its significance currently eludes me . . . but I think it might have something to do with this book . . . or the meaning of life. Whatever.

I elaborated greatly on the topic of code words and phrases in my story—words and phrases I had used that were later repeated. These repetitions, echoes, still figure prominently in my life. Only now I attribute these echoes to my being psychic.

Finally, I believe the sensation of déjà vu is directly related to psychic dreams. How can you remember something you are ostensibly seeing for the first time, unless you have already seen it in your mind, in your dreams?

Unscientific? Maybe. But the way I see it, either I am psychic or I *am* being followed, tapped, bugged, and so on. I know I prefer to consider myself psychic rather than paranoid. As a person with self-avowed psychic abilities, I may be deemed odd or eccentric, but at least I remain within the realm of sanity.

So, theory number two is that paranoia is a direct result of extreme psychic ability coupled with a logic that denies that psychic ability *is* real.

Why do visual hallucinations occur? My third theory addresses this question.

In short, I think my perspective is different from the norm. In endeavoring to see the unseen, I look at objects from every possible angle, from a surreal point of view. I know artists, painters, do this all of the time. But manics go too far. Because we *must* see the unseen—because we must make the necessary connections so that our notion of oneness remains intact—we create it in our minds and it becomes visible only to us. Our perspective, then, goes from real to surreal to unreal.

My fourth theory addresses auditory hallucinations. Part of this theory is that I think the nonsensical voices are the products of our memories. These voices are snippets of phrases we have heard at some point in the past, in no particular order. The other part of this theory relates to conversational voices. If we mentally separate ourselves from our voices, as I did with Carol, conversations can ensue. At this juncture I honestly believe that these conversational voices were me talking to me, another part of me. The child in me? Maybe. Or perhaps these voices were from a higher me and were revealing some of the wisdom buried deep within my subconscious.

My fifth theory addresses the confused emotions that accompany manic-depressive breakdowns. Perhaps the saddest idea that I entertained while psychotic was the notion that love and hate were one and the same. Both express passion, and to be passionate about someone or something is to care. And if you care, do you really hate?

I have always felt that hate is "the absence of caring." So for me, love and hate bled into one and resulted in terrible confusion. In loving my family, did I in fact hate them? Did I even know what love is? Ultimately, I decided that love and hate are mutually exclusive; my mental health could not withstand any blurred relationship between the two. My fifth theory, then, is that confused emotions are the result of blurred interpretations of love and hate, of good and evil.

These next two theories break from the preceding theories in that they address possible *causes* of chemical imbalances. I stress that these theories are completely unscientific, but I include them nonetheless as they have merit to me.

My sixth theory relates to the brain and its two sides. The right side of the brain is said to be the artistic side; and the left, the logical side. In my story I often state that I was as logical as I was crazy. All of my life, I have continually exercised both sides of the brain. Art and logic have always been equally important to me. So I wonder whether mania could be the result of overtaxing your brain's capabilities; that is, my theory is that we were designed to be good at either art or logic, but not both.

My seventh and final theory addresses another possible cause of mania. I contend that mania exists when the human brain and body cannot withstand the mind's capabilities. The mind—the soul—joins the human body through the brain. The mind, when free of the body, has limitless capabilities. Manics go beyond using their brains; they use their minds. My final theory, therefore, is that the mind and the brain are distinct entities and that prolonged usage of the mind results in mania.

I have no real theories regarding depression, except to say that it starts early on in life and grows over time. I believe the depression from which I suffered was both chemical and psychological. Indeed, I believe that the treatment of depression can be successful only if both the chemical and psychological aspects are addressed. To me, the best and only way out of psychological depression is to examine your life with all of its ups and downs, and let go of the downs. Learning, in my experience, is very effective in healing depression, as is music.

I want to get where I'm going
'Cause I've been where I'm at. (There's a bit of Newfie in me after all.)

To know all, one must experience both sanity and insanity, and have the sanity to know the difference!

Mom always said I was a "know-it-all."

Around the Block

My spirit's free—it's flying
To places, distant, calling me
To share the beauty of their jewels
And when I search I find that
The game's the same, no matter, but
I like to play by my own rules

A song is wailing—it screams
Of love, you know, sometimes it seems
The notes ring true but no one hears
But still I fly, it scares me
To think of those who never try
To reach the stars, grounded by fears

And I've been everywhere
Around the block—a moment here
But I could not wait for you
'Cause time you waste is time you lose

In shadowed dreams I've seen a
New color scheme, it screams of
Blue, black and green, they seem so new.

Song "Around the Block" © 1990, J. M. Knudsen

End Note

In the late '80s I noticed a beautiful porcelain doll in a store in my neighborhood. I remember going to that store with my mom and mentioning to her that had I the money, I would buy that doll. Well, Christmas morning I opened up my present—and discovered my porcelain doll.

The doll is beautiful. She is clad in silver and pearls. Her face is porcelain white, her makeup gold. There are teardrops painted below her eyes. She is also musical. When you wind her up, the theme from the movie *Love Story* plays and she sways to the music. Clearly my beautiful porcelain doll inspired me. Indeed, I came upon the title of my book when I first wrote a line that included the words "porcelain doll." I knew instantly that was my title. I knew instantly that I was the doll.

My very first line in the preface, "So . . . where do I begin," is actually derived from the opening lyrics to the *Love Story* theme. Interestingly, I had not listened to the doll in years. I was more than halfway through the book when I noticed this oneness.

Yes, my doll inspired me. God does work in mysterious ways.

One final note: we have been politically correct in renaming the illness manic depression, "bipolar disorder."

Good afternoon ladies and gentlemen. This is your captain speaking. We are presently cruising at an altitude of 32,000 feet. I would ask that you remain seated with your seat belts fastened as we are experiencing a slight bipolar disorder.

And now you can see why I still prefer the term "manic depression."

Once upon a time

In a land of snow and fire

There lived a girl who
reached the stars

And climbed a little higher

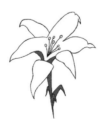

Order Form

The Porcelain Doll
Janet Knudsen
ISBN: 1-894372-32-8
$19.95 CAN / $15.00 US

The following discounts apply for orders of 10 or more copies:
Bookstores and Retail Accounts: 40%+
Wholesalers: 46%+
Educational Institutions: 20%
Public Libraries: 20%
Medical practitioners/corporate clients: 40%

All orders must include applicable sales taxes.

Allow $3.00 S&H for single copies and $5.00 for multiple copies

Quantity	Unit Price	Amount
	$19.95 CAN	
	$15.00 US	
_____		_____
Applicable Discounts		_____
Applicable Sales Taxes		_____
Shipping and Handling		_____
TOTAL		_____

QUICKFAX or
e-mail your order:
Fax: (506) 632-4009
E-mail: dcpub@fundy.net

DreamCatcher Publishing
105 Prince William Street
Saint John, NB, Canada E2L 2B2
Web: www.dreamcatcherbooks.ca